REASONABLE RISK
Alcohol in Perspective

Marjana Martinic and Barbara Leigh

BRUNNER-ROUTLEDGE

NEW YORK AND HOVE

Published in 2004 by
Brunner-Routledge
29 West 35th Street
New York, NY 10001
www.brunner-routledge.com

Published in Great Britain by
Brunner-Routledge
27 Church Road
Hove, East Sussex
BN3 2FA
www.brunner-routledge.co.uk

Brunner-Routledge is an imprint of the Taylor & Francis Group.
Printed in the United States of America on acid-free paper.

10 9 8 7 6 5 4 3 2 1

Library of Congress Cataloging-in-Publication Data

Martinic, Marjana.
    Reasonable risk : alcohol in perspective / by Marjana Martinic and Barbara Leigh.
       p. cm. — (International Center for Alcohol Policies series on alcohol in society)
    Includes bibliographical references and index.
    ISBN 0-415-94636-0
    1. Alcoholism—Social aspects. 2. Alcoholism—Risk factors. 3. Risk perception. 4. Risk assessment. 5. Risk management. I. Leigh, Barbara (Barbara C.) II. Title. III. Series on alcohol in society.
    HV5035.M374 2004
    362.292—dc22

                                                              2004043575

Contents

Acknowledgments

The authors would like to acknowledge the following individuals, without whom this book would not have been possible: Joanne Freeman, Tony Pyle, and Daniya Tamendarova for their tireless and meticulous editorial work; Dwight Heath for generously sharing his experience and wisdom; Wilson Acuda, Nick Alexander, Jan Buckingham, Troy Duster, Sietze Montijn, Ron Simpson, and Paul Slovic for their guidance in shaping the book; George Zimmar for his support and flexible definition of deadlines; and especially Marcus Grant for his vision and difficult questions that guided the writing of this book.

STATEMENT OF SUPPORT

Reasonable Risk was produced with the support of the International Center for Alcohol Policies (ICAP). ICAP is a not-for-profit organization whose mission is to promote understanding of the role of alcohol in society and to help reduce the abuse of alcohol worldwide, and to encourage dialogue and pursue partnerships with the beverage alcohol industry, the public health community and others interested in alcohol policy. ICAP is supported by major international producers of beverage alcohol. The views expressed in this book do not necessarily represent those of ICAP or of its sponsoring companies.

Setting the Stage

"Without numbers, there are no odds and probabilities; without odds and probabilities, the only way to deal with risk is to appeal to the gods and the fates. Without numbers, risk is wholly a matter of gut."

Bernstein, Against the Gods, 1996, p. 23

We cannot escape the hazards that surround us. Great or small, they are ubiquitous. An element of danger is present in virtually every human activity, whether it is driving to work in morning rush hour traffic, stepping off a curb to cross the street, or living in regions where infectious diseases abound. Hazards are inherent in our environment (e.g., acid rain and pollution, a thinning ozone layer, and industrial waste) and in our lifestyles (e.g., sexual behavior, smoking, extreme sports, diet, and exercise). We face all these hazards, voluntarily or involuntarily, as we are exposed to the world around us. Even the most mundane everyday activities may be fraught with danger (Figure 1).

The predictability of these hazards (e.g., the potential dangers that may affect us directly) lies at the heart of what we know as risk. As a concept, risk helps us to justify misfortune and frightening events and to explain deviations from what we consider the norm. It enables us to cope more effectively with uncertainty and with the things we fear, do not understand, or cannot control. The concept of risk is arguably one of the strategies developed by societies to deal with danger, with threats to human life, and with the unknown. Without these coping strategies, we would be forced to relinquish all sense of control and put ourselves at the mercy of fate; with them, we have a fighting chance of maintaining our equilibrium.

It is curious to note that although we willingly embrace some risks, we immediately reject others. Some risks are considered "good," and others are

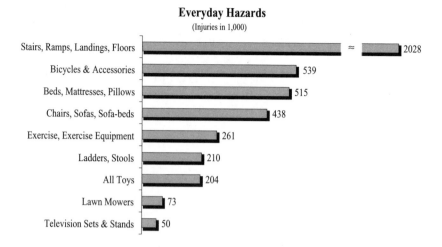

FIGURE 1. Estimated number of injuries from consumer products in the United States in 2002 (per 1000). *Source:* U.S. Consumer Product Safety Commission, 2003.

terrifying. What calculations do we, consciously or subconsciously, apply in each of these cases? How can we account for the often profoundly divergent ways in which the same potential hazards are viewed by different people—as too risky by some, as perfectly acceptable by others? How we weigh one hazard against another and evaluate the potential costs of certain situations against their potential benefits lies at the heart of our lifestyles, and frequently determines the luxury we have to engage in activities such as sports, adventure, and travel. For many of us, it can be argued that our preoccupation with risk is symptomatic of a modern and affluent world. When we run out of threats to worry about, we create new ones. Although this may be an exaggeration, understanding how risks to individuals and populations are viewed and managed may help put some of our own worries into perspective.

Within the broader context of general risk, this book examines the aura of risk surrounding alcohol consumption. Alcohol has been an integral part of many cultures around the world for thousands of years—as elixir, palliative, food, medicine, intoxicant, social lubricant, and ritual aid. Most people who drink are motivated largely by the prospect that they will enjoy it. For some, drinking provides an outlet, offers pleasure, and even provides benefit within a healthy lifestyle. For others, alcohol consumption can represent considerable risk to health and well-being.

Hazards are present not only for drinkers, but also for those around them, and even for society as a whole. In many ways, the risks inherent in drinking are no different from those we willingly encounter as part of other activities, including skiing, mountain climbing, overeating, riding a motorcycle, or driving a car. Yet, how we view the saliency of these potential hazards and the inherent riskiness of alcohol consumption varies considerably across individuals, groups, and even entire cultures. Finding the appropriate niche for alcohol in our panoply of risks is a complicated and challenging task.

The myriad ways in which we perceive the risks of alcohol consumption and the elements that shape this perception are addressed in Chapter 1. Depending on who we are and the circumstances surrounding our actions, we are likely to view the same risks in a different light. Although some risks may seem to us insignificant and trivial, a price we will gladly pay for the perceived benefits to be derived, others may seem daunting and not worth the cost. How we as individuals respond to risk may also be quite different from how we respond at the societal level. In general, we tend to view ourselves as less likely to actually suffer adverse consequences, not only from drinking, but also from virtually any potential hazard, than other people and the population in general. A wide disparity also exists between personal, "gut" reactions to risk and what the experts and their statistics tell us.

Culture is one of the most significant influences in how we view risks in lifestyle choices, including the consumption of alcohol. How we drink, how much we drink, and whether we drink at all are behaviors that are closely linked to general cultural attitudes about the role of alcohol in society and the acceptability of various drinking behaviors. Chapter 2 examines the components of culture that influence the construction of risk and help define what we consider normative behavior and its deviations. This chapter also discusses ways to maintain boundaries and minimize the potential for harm. In addition, it examines the place of alcohol within society and our shifting perspectives on its intrinsic risk.

The highly technical world of risk assessment and measurement provides fodder for Chapter 3. A foray into the role of research in risk assessment offers the reader an overview of what is involved in interpreting studies on risk, and what the results and related scientific jargon mean. *Relative risk, odds ratio,* and *cohort study* are terms that, for most of us, might as well be in a foreign language. Chapter 3 explains the way in which studies concerning risk are structured and how the resulting information affects us as individuals.

The ability to make our way through the language of risk equips us with some of the skills necessary to understand information that may reach us from a variety of sources. Much of what we are told about certain risks comes from those who, by virtue of their role in society, are in some way responsible for our safety and well-being. Other information on risk, however, comes from sources that may apply different prisms to the communication of risk information. Chapter 4 examines how those of us at the receiving end of risk information strive to make sense of what we are told. It also looks at those responsible for communicating risk information, the roles they play, and the qualifications that allow them to assume these roles, as well as other factors that influence what and how much information they share with the public.

Dealing with risk, based on information given to us and our own experience and perceptions, involves day-to-day decision making. It is important to understand that managing risks does not necessarily mean reducing them. When we manage risks in our lives, we are making decisions about our behaviors and weighing their respective risks and benefits. As with any other aspect of daily life, the decision of whether or not to drink beverage alcohol represents the balance of such calculations. Chapter 5 explores how we weigh the equation and whether the outcomes of drinking are acceptable to us as individuals and as a society.

The societal implications of risk management are addressed in the final chapter, which looks at the role of risk in the formulation of policy. Chapter 6 focuses specifically on how alcohol policies are developed within the context of individual and societal responsibility and the entities that are involved in the formulation of these policies. It examines the roles of all "players" involved in policy development, including government, nongovernmental organizations, the private sector, and society in general. It proposes an integrative approach based on partnership and risk minimization to develop effective approaches to alcohol policies.

This volume is not intended as a textbook. It does not purport to be a scientific treatise on risk that is written for experts and those engaged in alcohol research. Instead, using scientific evidence as a base, it seeks to offer the educated "layman" a lucid and comprehensible explanation of the elements that contribute to how we view risks in general, particularly risks associated with alcohol. It also offers insight into how we assess and attempt to manage the risks confronting us.

Drinking beverage alcohol is relatively common in most societies, an activity that carries the potential for harm in a variety of situations and contexts. That much is incontrovertible and must be acknowledged. At the same time, when dealing with risks associated with drinking or any other behavior, it is worthwhile to take a step back and examine where these risks fall within the context of other risks. The risks that face us have a hierarchy. Some are life threatening, while others are but an inconvenience. If we are to understand the risks that confront us and hope to manage them effectively, it is important that we comprehend how they fit into the overall order of things and why they concern us in the way they do.

REFERENCES

U.S. Consumer Product Safety Commission (2003, Fall). NEISS Data Highlights — 2002. *Consumer Product Safety Review, 8(2)*, 3–7.

Chapter 1

Keeping an Eye Out: Our Perceptions of Risk

It worries me greatly, but the facts don't seem to help much. People just have an inappropriate sense of what is dangerous. They get overly upset about minor problems. If you translate the weight and time it takes a laboratory rat to develop bladder cancer to a 200-pound man drinking Fresca, it comes out to about two bathtubs full each day. People dropped Fresca in a minute, but they continue to smoke.

Surgeon General C. Everett Koop quoted in the
Los Angeles Times, *May 9, 1989 (Taylor, 1990)*

In our modern world, risks and judgments about risks present a paradox: People today, on average, are healthier and safer than ever before, but, at the same time, they feel more vulnerable and are more concerned about risk (Keeney, 1994; Skolbekken, 1995; Slovic, 1997). Much of this apprehension springs from new technologies and environmental hazards, although concerns also exist about health behaviors as well as the risks associated with the foods we eat and the beverages we drink.

High levels of perceived risk, from technology or from other aspects of our lives, may spring from several sources including:

Our increasing ability to measure tiny amounts of toxic substances.
Our growing reliance on technologies, which can be very dangerous if they fail.
Our memory of catastrophic mishaps such as Bhopal, India, and Chernobyl, Ukraine.
Increasing (and highly publicized) litigation over risk problems.

A growing sense that we should have control over most risks in our lives, whether personal or societal (Slovic, 1997).

Whatever the reason for these high levels of concern, studies of risk perception "attempt to understand this paradox and to understand why it is that our perceptions are so often at variance with what the experts say we should be concerned about" (Slovic, 1997, p. 233). In this chapter, we examine how people perceive the risks and benefits of various activities, substances, and technologies. We briefly outline research on risk perception in general, and then we focus on risk perception as it applies to alcohol consumption.

APPROACHES TO RISK PERCEPTION

Modern research on risk perception has evolved in recent years, "*from* an emphasis on 'public misperceptions,' with a tendency to treat all deviations from expert estimates as products of ignorance or stupidity; *via* empirical investigation of what actually concerns people and why; *to* approaches which stress that public reactions to risk often have a rationality of their own, and that 'expert' and 'lay' perspectives should inform each other as part of a two-way process" (Bennett, 1999).

Technical Risk

Emphasizing public misperceptions of risk reflects the traditional dichotomy between the risk judgments of experts and the public. From a "pure engineering" view (Fisk, 1999), probabilities of harm can be calculated from hard data, and the results can be seen as reflecting "objective" risk. This "technical risk" represents both the probability of an untoward event and the magnitude of its consequences (Kasperson, 1992). For example, although some risks have a low probability of occurrence and very severe consequences (e.g., death from a nuclear power plant accident), others have a high probability of occurrence and somewhat benign consequences (e.g., getting a cold).

This so-called "objective" risk does not map well onto people's subjective impressions of those risks. Popular books (Glassner, 1999; Paling & Paling, 1994; Ross, 1999), media reports, and empirical research provide a litany of examples showing that the risk judgments of laypeople are at variance with what we are told by experts. For example, although people express great concern about nuclear power and toxic chemicals, which pose improbable risks, they don't appear to be as concerned with the risks of motor vehicles and obesity, which, in fact, cause much more damage. People also underestimate the frequency of common high-probability causes of death (e.g., emphysema or diabetes) and overestimate the likelihood of low-probability causes that are more dramatic or sensational (e.g., botulism, tornadoes, and shark attacks) (Lichtenstein, Slovic, Fischhoff, Layman, & Combs, 1978; Spencer & Crossen, 2003).

The problem with "objective" measures of risk is that they are not objective; they reflect the judgment of the scientists who produce them. Risk estimates are based on theoretical models that are constructed from various assumptions. They depend on judgments at all stages: deciding how to define the problem, which consequences to include, how to estimate the exposures, how to integrate results from existing studies, and how to extrapolate information from different domains (e.g., generalizing from animal research to health effects on humans). Scientists are subject to errors and biases, as well as to monetary and political pressures. Thus, risk estimates are inherently subjective (Fischhoff, Slovic, & Lichtenstein, 1983; Freudenburg, 1988; Slovic, 1999).

Even somewhat simple measurements, such as numbers of fatalities, incorporate judgments and values. Although the end point appears well defined—either you're dead or you're not—the choice of how the measurement is obtained is a subjective judgment. We can measure mortality from auto crashes by deaths per 1 million people, per mile driven, per auto trip taken, or per automobile on the road; or we can base our measurements on the lowered life expectancy among the driving population. Our choice can make a difference in how the risk is perceived or evaluated. It also reflects our values. If we summarize a risk as reduction in life expectancy, we are treating young deaths as more important than older deaths; if we count all fatalities equally, we are treating quick deaths in the same manner as painful, lingering deaths. Treating deaths differently or treating them as equivalent are both value judgments (Keeney, 1994; Slovic, 1999).

We can also choose measurements in ways that highlight either risk or safety. Between 1950 and 1970, the number of accidental deaths among miners per ton of mined coal decreased, but the number of accidental deaths per employee increased (Slovic, 1999). Did coal mining become more or less safe in those 20 years? The answer would probably depend on whether one's sympathies lie with labor or with the mine owners.

Moreover, there is great uncertainty and error in quantifying risks and benefits, uncertainties that "often defy systematic analysis and preclude scientific consensus" (Nelkin, 1989, p. 100). Both scientists and the public often underestimate these uncertainties (Freudenburg, 1988). Even fundamental physical measurements, such as the speed of light, differ by huge magnitudes: The 1984 estimate of the speed of light falls outside the standard error for all the values reported between 1930 and 1970 (Freudenburg, 1988). Measures of risk carry similar uncertainties. "Although there are actual risks, nobody knows what they are" (Fischhoff et al. 1983, p. 236).

The objective/subjective distinction rests on an assumption that "evaluating risk is a technical matter to be resolved by developing better, more accurate scientific information; that there is an optimal way to characterize risk that reflects an underlying consensus among experts; that people fear technology because they are poorly informed or fail to understand the nature of risk; that they are misled by exaggerated media reports, or hold basically irrational, anti-science views" (Nelkin, 1989, p. 99).

The assumption that the experts are correct and the public is misguided is a false distinction that engenders disrespect between the parties involved (Fischhoff et al., 1983). As Gigerenzer (2000, p. 237) notes, "The political implications of this view are not hard to see: given the message that ordinary citizens are unable to estimate uncertainties and risks, one might conclude that a government would be well advised to keep these nitwits out of important decisions regarding new technologies and environmental risks."

Playing up the discrepancies between the judgments of experts and laypeople highlights the tendency of the technical literature on risk to purvey an "ill-masked contempt for laypeople's lack of what is learned to be 'appropriate' or 'correct' knowledge about risk. Laypeople are often portrayed as responding 'unscientifically' to risk, using inferior and unsophisticated sources of knowledge such as 'intuition'" (Lupton, 1999, p. 19). Thus, by considering the experts' views of risk as scientific and objective, laypeople's concerns can be dismissed as the product of irrational emotions and biases.

Lay Concepts of Risk

The discrepancies between technical risk estimates by experts and people's risk perceptions set the stage for social scientists to study the aspects of potential risks that most concern us. Risk perception among laypeople includes many aspects not measured by the technical approach. It includes values such as emotional distress, disruption of social relationships, attitudes toward authority that may foster mistrust, political priorities, and cultural expectations (Nelkin, 1989).

Cognitive psychologists, who have conducted scores of studies in which people are questioned about their perceptions, attitudes, and judgments of risk, have spearheaded research on these experiential aspects of risk perception. By studying public perceptions of the risk of numerous phenomena, including environmental risks, technological innovations, and health issues, these researchers have uncovered the ways in which people judge real-life risks, taking into account not only the technical "facts," but also personal values, societal goals, and emotional responses. Whereas "specialists" see risk in terms of quantitative outcomes, such as mortality, nonspecialists incorporate qualitative considerations into their judgments (National Research

Council, 1996). For example, two different risks might have the same absolute probability of mortality, and, therefore, these risks might be judged as equally risky in the technical sense. Most people judging these risks would also consider the manner of death in the risk equation, however, assigning greater risk to a phenomenon that might result in a more lingering or unpleasant death.

Whereas scientists formulate risk in terms of effects on populations, laypeople tend to reframe the information in terms of personal risk: What does this mean for my family and me? (Bennett, 1999; National Research Council, 1996). People distinguish between the risks that they think are important on a societal level and the problems that affect them personally. For example, if people report being concerned about crime, they may mean that they think crime is a serious social problem, not that crime is personally threatening in their own lives (Weinstein, 1989).

Integrating Expert and Lay Perspectives

The disjuncture in risk studies between "technical" and "social" or "perceptual" analysis of hazards (Freudenburg, 1988) leads to conflicts stemming from the differences in definitions between experts and laypeople. Although experts define risk in a technical way, the public's view is more complex, incorporating value considerations such as equity, catastrophic potential, and controllability (Slovic, 1992, p. 150). Because laypeople incorporate value considerations into their judgments, citations of "actual" risks by experts often don't change people's perceptions of risk very much.

Current thinking on risk perception acknowledges both aspects of risk: the technical, which studies and defines probabilities of harm, and the experiential, which reflects the aspects of risk about which the public cares. The public's perceptions, or intuitive risk assessments, differ in their assumptions based on scientists' models; however, these intuitive assessments do include elements of rationality (National Research Council, 1996). "The public is not irrational. The public is influenced by emotion and affect in a way that is both simple and sophisticated. So are scientists. The public is influenced by worldviews, ideologies, and values. So are scientists, particularly when they are working at the limits of their expertise" (Slovic, 1999, p. 699).

WHAT SHAPES OUR PERCEPTIONS OF RISK?

The "Personality" of Risk

A series of studies by cognitive psychologists has identified aspects of various hazards that lead to differences in how their risks are perceived (Slovic,

1992). Every hazard has a pattern of qualities that is related to perceived risk. These attributes can help explain why some activities (e.g., nuclear power) arouse so much more public opposition than others (e.g., motorcycle riding) that cause more fatalities (National Research Council, 1996). These attributes can be viewed as reflecting a "personality" of risk, meaning that some forms of risk engender much anxiety and alarm regardless of the scientific estimates of their seriousness.

The following categories for the "personality" of risk have been proposed:

Imposed or involuntary risks vs. chosen risks. People make a strong distinction between chosen and imposed risks. "People who knowingly take risks do to themselves what they wouldn't let others do to them" (Imperato & Mitchell, 1985, p. 1). Involuntary risks challenge our personal autonomy and are viewed more negatively than risks we choose (Bennett, 1999). In reality, the distinction isn't all that clear; there are few truly chosen risks and also few truly imposed risks (Imperato & Mitchell, 1985). In particular, there is disagreement about the voluntariness of technologies. For example, each ride in a car might be voluntary, but, in the larger sense, the alternatives are fictitious in modern society (Fischhoff et al., 1983).

Unfamiliar vs. familiar. We interact with many familiar risks daily: driving or riding in a car, using a household appliance, or drinking beverage alcohol. In contrast, such hazards as toxic chemicals and nuclear power are technologies with which most people have no personal experience and toward which they have more negative attitudes.

Controllable vs. uncontrollable. This dimension is similar (but not identical) to the voluntary-involuntary dimension described previously. A sense of personal control over our lives is important to us, and hazards that we cannot control are particularly unacceptable.

Man-made vs. naturally occurring. Although man-made and naturally occurring phenomena can have equally catastrophic consequences (e.g., an industrial accident and a flood may both take hundreds of lives), we express more distaste for man-made problems.

Dreaded vs. not dreaded. Some causes of death arouse particular dread. For example, a lingering, painful death from a poorly understood cause, such as radiation sickness, would instill greater fear than a death from a more familiar cause, such as a heart attack.

Hazards are also viewed negatively to the extent that they are seen as inequitably distributed in society, immune to precautions, poorly understood by science, causing hidden or irreversible damage, or threatening to future generations. These "fright factors" represent defensible value judgments, reflecting our beliefs about how society is and should be, our relationship with nature, and the benefits and disadvantages of technology (Bennett, 1999).

Many of these dimensions are related to each other. For example, hazards seen as voluntary tend also to be judged as controllable. Slovic (1987) has reduced many of these attributes to two dimensions. The first dimension reflects whether the risk has elements of dread, uncontrollability, and fatal consequences; the second dimension reflects whether the risk is known and understood vs. unknown and unobservable. Figure 1.1, which represents more than 30,000 individual judgments about risks, shows the positioning of risks associated with a number of technologies and hazards in this two-dimensional space. Nuclear technologies, including nuclear power and nuclear weapons, are unknown and dreaded, as are many chemicals. At the other end of the spectrum are familiar and controllable risks, such as alcohol, smoking, and swimming pools.

People's perceptions of the riskiness of a phenomenon are related to its position in this two-dimensional space. Technologies, behaviors, and elements that are regarded as more uncontrollable and more unfamiliar are considered more risky, while familiar and understandable elements are considered less risky—even though many of these more familiar risks result in a greater number of fatalities. In addition, the more dread and uncontrollability attributed to a hazard, the more people want to see stricter regulation to reduce the risk. Here again, we see the distinction between technical risk, based on probability of adverse outcomes, and experiential risk, which incorporates notions of dread and uncontrollability (Slovic, Finucane, Peters, & MacGregor, 2002).

Nuclear power risks offer an example of extreme positions in this model. Although the 1979 accident at the Three Mile Island nuclear reactor near Harrisburg, Pennsylvania, resulted in no deaths, it produced costly social impacts. The accident increased opposition to nuclear power and led to stricter regulation of the nuclear industry. Such an accident in a system that is unfamiliar or poorly understood can be interpreted as a signal that the system might cause further, possibly catastrophic, mishaps. In contrast, an accident in a familiar system (e.g., a plane crash), although devastating to the victims and their family and friends, might cause relatively little disturbance to the public (Slovic, 1987).

Optimistic Bias

Although we often think of adolescents as possessing an illusory sense of invulnerability, in reality this tendency is present in all of us. People tend to rate the chances that something bad will happen to them as much lower than they rate chances that such a thing will happen to other people. For example, people rate themselves as better drivers than others (Svenson, Fischhoff, & MacGregor, 1985), see themselves as less likely to be hurt by consumer

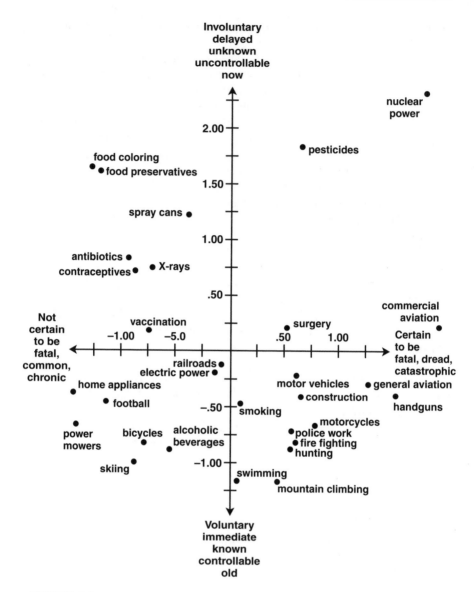

FIGURE 1.1. Characteristics of hazards on risk dimensions. Adapted with permission from Slovic, P. (1987). Perception of risk. *Science, 236*(4799), 280–285. Copyright 1987 by the American Association for the Advancement of Science. Reprinted with permission.

products (Slovic, Fischhoff, & Lichtenstein, 1982), and view themselves as less likely to be the victim of a crime (Perloff & Fetzer, 1986).

This tendency also applies to a wide range of life events, health outcomes, and safety hazards, including food poisoning, auto accidents, poison ivy, sunstroke, gum disease, cancer, drug addiction, and heart disease. Even people who clearly engage in a health-compromising behavior show such a bias. Smokers perceive themselves to be at lower risk for lung cancer than other smokers (Slovic, 2000a), and homosexual men who engage in unsafe sex see themselves as less likely to contract HIV than other gay men (van der Pligt, Otten, & Richard, 1993). In general, although people do not see themselves as invulnerable to harm, they are "unrealistically optimistic" about their susceptibility to harm. This bias applies across age, sex, education, and occupational status and differs across a range of hazards. The extent of the bias is greater for the following kinds of outcomes (Weinstein, 1989):

Outcomes that are perceived as preventable or controllable by personal action. If we admit that we are vulnerable to outcomes that we could prevent, we threaten our self-esteem by implying that we lack self-control or coping ability. The more preventable or controllable the hazard, the stronger the tendency to claim below-average risk (Weinstein, 1989).

Outcomes that are stigmatized. Outcomes that are embarrassing or generally disapproved of also threaten self-esteem. These outcomes, including alcohol dependence, drug addiction, and sexually transmitted diseases, are also particularly susceptible to optimistic bias.

Outcomes that are low in probability. Most bad things that can happen to people happen very rarely, and many people never experience them. Our lack of experience with a problem may make it seem unlikely to happen, and because we don't consider that it's also unlikely for others, we may conclude that our risk is below average. For example, even the poorest drivers drive a lot without having accidents, and any accidents that they hear about happen to others. Thus, in the experience of these drivers, they are safer than average (Slovic, Fischhoff, & Lichtenstein, 2000).

Perceptual Biases: Availability

Assessing risk is a complex task. We have to amass information on the probabilities of harm and on the severity of outcomes and somehow integrate that information. Many cognitive psychologists claim that our cognitive abilities are not always up to the task. Some concepts are very difficult for people; for example, we have difficulty understanding very low probabilities and cumulative probabilities.

Instead of weighing and measuring all the information, psychologists suggest that we rely on *heuristics*, or rules of thumb, to reduce complex tasks to simpler judgments. In many cases, these heuristics lead to accurate judgments, but they can also lead to systematic errors. To judge the frequency or probability (or risk) of an outcome or event, we often make judgments based on how easily instances of the event come to mind. The easier it is to remember or imagine an event, the higher the perceived probability that it will occur. This rule of thumb for probability judgments is called the *availability heuristic* (Tversky & Kahneman, 1974). Using such a heuristic can lead to accurate estimates, given that examples of more frequent occurrences are easier to bring to mind than examples of less frequent occurrences.

Our ability to recall or imagine events, however, is affected by not only the frequency and probability of those events. We are more likely to bring to mind events that stand out because of their distinctiveness, emotional content, or recency, whether or not those events actually occur with the most frequency. If we judge an occurrence as more probable because it comes to mind readily, we will then view these distinctive, sensational events as occurring more frequently than they really do. Even imagining a hypothetical outcome, be it winning a contest or contracting a disease, leads people to believe that the outcome is more likely to happen.

An example of the workings of the availability heuristic in risk perception comes from a study in which people estimated the frequency of 41 causes of death in the U.S., from homicide and motor vehicle accidents to botulism, tornadoes, and electrocution (Slovic, Fischhoff, & Lichtenstein, 1979). Although most people ordered the causes of death correctly (i.e., they judged the frequency of heart disease as greater than homicide and greater than tornadoes), they overestimated the frequency of causes of death that were particularly sensational and visible. For example, people estimated that botulism (outbreaks of which are reported in the news media), which kills fewer than 10 people per year, was responsible for more than 500 deaths per year.

The Media

Several commentators have suggested that one reason our perceptions of risk are unrealistic is that the media provide sensational coverage of outcomes that are actually uncommon (Glassner, 1999). Examples of disproportionate coverage, from shark attacks to child kidnappings, are easy to find. (It is interesting that journalists are both promoters and debunkers of popular fears, and, as will be discussed in Chapter 4 on communicating risks, doubters of scientific research on risk.)

The effects of media reports on risk perception provide a real-world example of the availability heuristic previously discussed. The more we are confronted with information about a risk, the more likely that risk will come to mind, making it appear more likely to happen. For example, a study of press coverage of the U.S. "War on Drugs" in the mid- to late-1980s showed that press coverage describing drug use as a crisis could explain the changes in public opinion about the drug problem in the U.S. This sequence would not be problematic if media reports accurately reflected the severity of social problems; however, for many problems, the reportage is inaccurate and sensational.

Note that the availability heuristic implies that discussing risks in the news, even without sensational or exaggerated coverage, leads to an increased perception of risk. For example, a study of perceived risks of electric and magnetic fields from electric blankets and power lines demonstrated that these risks were perceived initially as relatively low. Study participants were then given information about research on the health effects of such fields. The information indicated that studies had been done on the topic, but that the research had shown no human health effects of these fields. When asked again about their perception of these risks, study participants rated the risk as greater than they had before receiving the information, even though the information did not link electric and magnetic fields with increased risk to human health (Morgan, 1985).

Affect, Emotion, and Stigma

Recent research has examined the role of *affect* as an orienting mechanism for risk perception. Affect, a positive or negative evaluative feeling about something, is automatic (i.e., there are just some things that we like and others that we don't like). Often, we have immediate affective or "gut" reactions to things—reactions that are not based on any cognitive or perceptual information and that can guide our subsequent judgments (Zajonc, 1980, p. 155). According to an affective model, this primary evaluative reaction guides our perceptions of risks and benefits. As a result, when people like something, they see it as having high benefit and low risk; when they dislike something, they judge the benefits to be low and the risks to be high. In a series of studies testing this model, Slovic and colleagues (Finucane, Alhakami, Slovic, & Johnson, 2000; Slovic, Finucane, Peters, & MacGregor, 2002; Slovic, Finucane, Peters, & MacGregor, in press) demonstrated that altering the overall favorableness of a target also alters its perceived risks and benefits. For example, calling attention to the benefits of nuclear power reduced perceptions of the risk of nuclear power.

Affective responses can influence risk perception by stigmatizing a technology or health exposure. Stigma denotes something that is marked as deviant, undesirable, and outside the bounds of the "good" and "normal"; stigmatized objects are to be avoided and denigrated. Stigma is affect-based and can result in exaggerated negative perceptions, and it is closely associated with perceptions of risk.

For example, pollution from toxic substances can stigmatize entire geographical regions, such as Love Canal, New York, or Seveso, Italy, resulting in social and economic impacts on regions perceived as polluted (Slovic et al., 2002). Products can also become stigmatized: the intrauterine device (IUD) for birth control will remain stigmatized through its link with pelvic inflammatory disease; the ill-fated Ford Pinto will forever be associated with exploding gas tanks; and beef remains linked with mad cow disease. Manufacturers of certain products can also be stigmatized: Union Carbide's chemical plant disaster in Bhopal, India, has not been forgotten, nor has Exxon's oil spill in Alaska's Prince William Sound (Slovic, 1992). In a recent study of perceptions of the safety of the blood supply in the U.S. (Finucane, Slovic, & Mertz, 2000), survey respondents were asked about the perceived risk of the blood supply and about the images that they associated with blood transfusions. The concept of blood transfusion often evoked images of AIDS or HIV, and a substantial proportion of the respondents did not deem the blood supply safe, claiming they would not accept blood if hospitalized. Thus, although blood screening eliminated HIV risk from blood transfusions years ago, the initial link between HIV infection and blood transfusion appears to have stigmatized the blood supply and still leads to heightened concern about its risks.

THE PERCEIVED RISKS AND BENEFITS OF DRINKING

Many factors influence how we perceive the risks in the world around us, including risks that may be found in commonplace, everyday activities, in what we eat and drink, and how we lead our lives. Our perception of risks that may lie in the consumption of alcohol is no exception. Much of what we know about how people perceive the risks and benefits of drinking comes from research on *alcohol expectancies*—people's beliefs about the effects of alcohol on their behavior, moods, and emotions. A wealth of research shows that people hold a number of common expectancies about the behavioral and emotional effects of alcohol (see Critchlow, 1986, for a review). An expectancy, essentially an "if–then" statement about alcohol effects, is a cognitive representation of our past direct and indirect experiences with alcohol.

Folkloric conceptions of a link between alcohol use and behavioral and personality changes are thousands of years old. Descriptions of alcohol-induced disinhibition appear in writings of the Greeks and Romans and continue in literature, film, song, and a host of other cultural manifestations. People have believed for centuries that alcohol affects them in desirable ways, while at the same time believing that alcohol is a source of immorality, crime, and all manner of deviant behavior.

In the behavioral sciences, the recent focus on the cognitive and social aspects of drinking has led to a number of studies that have identified and examined the content of these beliefs, as listed in Table 1.1:

TABLE 1.1 Positive and Negative Expectancies about Alcohol Consumption

Positive Effects		Negative Effects	
Social	more social	Social	aggressive
	less shy		loss of control
	more talkative		loud, obnoxious
	enhanced sexual		stupid, foolish
	arousal or performance		
Physical	get drunk	Physical	hangover
	increase energy		pass out
Emotional	relax		sick, headache
	feel good	Emotional	angry
	forget problems		depressed
	relieve tension		ashamed, guilty
	reduce stress	Cognitive	impaired judgment
Fun	good time		less alert
	interesting		poor concentration
	consciousness		decreased motor skills
	alteration		
	fun, pleasure	Consequences	work problems
	happy		accident
	buzz		trouble with the law
	tastes good		trouble with family or friends

Surveys and interviews show that people expect largely positive effects from drinking. When people are asked to list the effects that alcohol has on them, they tend to list more positive than negative effects and to list the positive effects first (Gustafson, 1988, 1989; Leigh & Stacy, 1994). For example, in Roizen's (1983) analysis of a U.S. national survey, the most commonly reported effects (cited by 70–80% of respondents) were generally positive (i.e., friendly, talkative, romantic). Unpleasant effects such as feeling sick, aggressive, argumentative, sad, or mean were reported less frequently. Moreover, people viewed the positive effects as more likely to occur.

As an interesting aside, it was not the case that some people reported positive effects and others reported negative effects. Instead, people who reported any effects mentioned positive ones, and only as the number of effects experienced became larger were negative effects included. Thus, people reported no effects, positive effects, or both positive and negative effects; no one reported negative effects without positive effects.

Although both drinkers and nondrinkers share a set of alcohol expectancies, these beliefs are influenced by age, culture, beverage, and situation:

Age. Beliefs about the effects of alcohol are present in children before their first personal experience with alcohol (Christiansen,

Goldman, & Inn, 1982; Christiansen, Smith, Roehling, & Goldman, 1989; Miller, Smith, & Goldman, 1990). Children may acquire these beliefs through observation, vicarious learning, and assimilation of cultural stereotypes (Critchlow, 1986). Young children tend to have predominantly negative beliefs about alcohol (Aitken, 1978; Isaacs, 1977; Jahoda & Cramond, 1972; Johnson & Johnson, 1995; Spiegler, 1983), although some positive beliefs also exist (Christiansen et al., 1982; Christiansen et al., 1989; Miller et al., 1990). Once children start experimenting with alcohol in early puberty, expectancies start to shift from negative to positive (Aitken, 1978; Johnson & Johnson, 1995). These emerging positive expectancies become stronger during subsequent years of drinking (Aas, Leigh, Anderssen, & Jakobsen, 1998). Lang and Michalac (1990) suggest that younger children's negative expectancies may reflect the discouraging messages coming from parents and other authority figures, while older children may tend to rebel against these figures. Younger children may also expect alcohol to make adults' behavior aversive and erratic—frightening effects that undermine children's security. As children become more sophisticated and capable of tolerating unpredictability, they may find the effects of alcohol more appealing (Lang, Murray, & Pelham, 1984).

Cultural and historical influences. If alcohol expectancies are part of shared cultural understandings, then they should vary for different cultures during different periods of history. Most cross-cultural studies of alcohol expectancies suggest that although there are differences in the strength with which the beliefs are held, the content of expectancies is similar. In studies of expectancies in different ethnic groups in the U.S., white male college students believed more strongly than black male college students that alcohol would affect their behavior (Reese & Friend, 1994); Hispanics expected more effects of all kinds (both positive and negative) than non-Hispanic Americans (Marín, 1996; Marín, Posner, & Kinyon, 1993; Velez-Blasini, 1997); and Asian-American college students, despite their lighter drinking habits, expected more tension reduction than non-Asian students (O'Hare, 1995). In a study of beliefs about alcohol-induced aggression in 10 countries, Lindman and Lang (1994) found that American and French survey respondents had particularly strong beliefs that alcohol causes aggressive behavior, while Spanish respondents tended to fall on the other end of the scale.

Beverage type. Different positive and negative expectancies have also been associated with various types of alcohol beverages. Among young drinkers surveyed in Florida and Finland, wine elicited the most expectancy for positive effects, followed by mixed drinks, beer, and distilled spirits (Lang, Kaas, & Barnes, 1983; Lindman & Lang, 1986). Beer was associated with lethargy and sleepiness, wine with contentment and romance, mixed drinks with sociability, and distilled spirits with unpleasant consequences of heavy use, such as passing out and loss of memory. The "unique constellations of expectations" related to different beverages may arise from the "distinctive conditions, purposes, and levels of their typical consumption" (Lang et al., 1983). In addition, such beliefs are probably influenced by culture and the particular role of alcohol within a given society.

Situation. The effects that people expect from drinking vary across situations. For example, in Roizen's (1983) study, respondents rarely reported that they always experienced any effect from drinking. Even for the most commonly reported effects, 10% or fewer respondents reported experiencing the effect on every drinking occasion. Similarly, in studies that required respondents to rate the likelihood of an effect occurring, respondents showed an unwillingness to use the end points of the scale; instead, they tended to report that alcohol affected their behavior "some of the time" (Leigh, 1987). In one such study (Leigh, 1987), many respondents made unsolicited comments that the effects they experienced when drinking depended on the situation. Roizen (1983) noted that "this observation would seem a nice demonstration that alcohol is not linked to its various effects in lockstep fashion in popular opinion but is instead regarded very much as a matter of the particularities of the drinking event. That most of us might agree that alcohol may help us to feel friendly does not, then, imply about common opinion that alcohol always or even usually will have this effect" (p. 241).

Both this lack of certainty and the unwillingness to consistently impute any specific effect to drinking suggest that people have a sense of the situational specificity of the effects of not only alcohol, but of any psychoactive substance. Laypeople already have a very good idea of what researchers have discovered: the effects of any substance are dependent on the setting in which it is consumed (Lettieri, Sayers, & Pearson, 1980).

Risk, Benefit, and Expectancy

As depicted in Figure 1.1, in comparison to other behaviors and technologies, alcohol falls among familiar, controllable, voluntary behaviors without catastrophic consequences. We might therefore expect that alcohol would be considered relatively low risk; however, other research using the same kinds of measurements suggests otherwise. In a study conducted in Sweden that assessed perceptions of risks and benefits of various medications, substances, and medical procedures (Slovic, 2000b), alcohol was perceived as quite low in benefits and high in risk, as plotted in Figure 1.2.

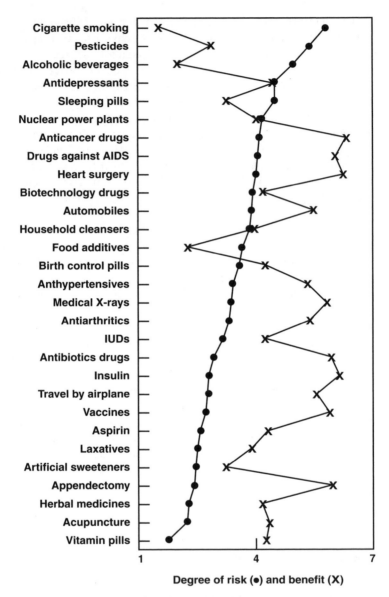

FIGURE 1.2. Rated risks and benefits of substances, technologies, and products. From Slovic, P. (2000b). The perception and management of therapeutic risk. In P. Slovic (Ed.), *The perception of risk* (pp. 246–263). London: Earthscan Publications. Reprinted with author's permission.

As Sjöberg (1998) notes, if it is assumed that people behave in accordance with the costs and benefits of their behavior, such findings make alcohol use incomprehensible. How do we reconcile these extreme risk perceptions with the fact that most drinkers report benefits from drinking (Mäkelä & Mustonen, 1988, 2000; Mustonen & Mäkelä, 1999)? For example, in Ontario in 1994, 14% of drinkers reported at least one alcohol-related problem, while 67% reported one or more benefits. The majority of drinkers (58%) reported that alcohol caused equivalent amounts of harm and good, 24% said that alcohol led to more good than harm, and only 10% said that it caused more harm than good (Bondy, 1996).

To reconcile these perceptions (that alcohol has great risk and little benefit) with findings from expectancy research (indicating that people experience good effects from alcohol) we can turn to three issues:

1. *Terminology.* In the Swedish study depicted in Figure 1.2, people were asked about the risks and benefits of several substances, including alcohol. "Benefits" may not be a word that people normally use to label the positive consequences of drinking (Sjöberg, 1998), especially in a context that also included questions about medications. That is, "benefit" may represent to people a discrete effect on health status; for example, antibiotics kill infections, sleeping pills help you sleep, and antidepressants cheer you up. The pleasant effects of alcohol, including sociability and relaxation, are more diffuse and less clearly related to human health.
2. *Enumeration of consequences.* Studies of risk perception often include measurements of several aspects of the hazards, as described previously. For example, people might be asked about the probability of harm along with aspects of dread, controllability, or equity; however, the actual consequences of the hazard are often left unstated. With alcohol, the potential consequences of drinking are quite extensive, as listed in Table 1.1. A single question about the "risks" and "benefits" of alcohol does not capture the variety of potential consequences, both positive and negative, of drinking.
3. *Personal vs. general risk.* In the Swedish study, as in other studies in this psychometric tradition, people were asked about their perceptions of the risk of various substances in general. As mentioned earlier, these general judgments about risk may represent concepts that people regard as serious social problems instead of problems to which they are personally susceptible. Cultural factors, such as Sweden's history of temperance and its tradition of explosive drinking, might lead that country's residents to view drinking as problematic on a societal level, with few benefits and much risk.

Beliefs in alcohol's essential malevolence usually come from people who are referring to the experiences of other people, not their own experiences, while expecting positive effects for themselves. Roizen (1983) noted that in a survey conducted in California, 62% of the respondents agreed that "drink can bring out the worst in people."

But however much these sorts of global estimates may suggest that American public opinion has embraced the notion that alcohol often can disinhibit or disrupt the drinker's behavior, it is well to remember that the respondent to these questions often has *somebody* else's, and not his own, drinking in mind. . . . Although almost two thirds of the population thought alcohol often brought out the worst in people, only about one in eight respondents reported being ashamed of something he himself did while drinking in the past year (Roizen, 1983, p. 237).

Similarly, when a sample of the Swedish population was asked about the causes of violence, the most common explanation given was alcohol and drugs; however, few respondents said that they themselves would become violent when drinking (Sjöberg, 1998). Other studies (Leigh, 1987; Rohsenow, 1983) show that people tend to see others as more likely to experience alcohol effects than they do—a tendency that is much stronger for negative than positive effects. Thus, perceptions of the risks of drinking reflect the optimistic bias discussed earlier in this chapter. Differences between general and personal risk may be influenced by self-esteem considerations, resulting in a tendency to view bad alcohol-related outcomes as happening to others, while claiming good outcomes for oneself (Agostinelli & Miller, 1994; Critchlow, 1986; Rohsenow, 1983).

Alternatively, these differences may signify that the bad things caused by drinking occur only rarely, and many people never experience them. If we never experience a certain outcome, we may see it as very unlikely to happen to us in the future. Although the positive aspects of drinking are widely known and shared, it is the negative behaviors that might be associated with alcohol, including violence and drunk driving, that make news. In reality, these negative consequences occur in only a small proportion of total drinking occasions, and most people have never experienced them. But given that these consequences are well known, people are aware that *somebody* is adversely affected by alcohol, although not themselves, and they perceive themselves as less likely than other people to experience these negative consequences.

As noted earlier in this chapter, unrealistic optimism tends to be greater for activities that are under a person's control. In a survey of Swedish citizens, this optimistic bias was particularly large for alcohol consumption, which was rated as one of the highest general risks and one of the smallest personal risks (Sjöberg, 1998). Other behaviors that are considered to be under personal control, such as smoking and contracting HIV, also exhibited large differences between general and personal risks.

SUMMARY

Psychological research on risk perception has demonstrated that laypeople have a more complex view of risk than do the scientists who compute risk measurements. Expert risk assessments rely on the probabilities of harm.

Although nonscientists can also make these assessments, they include other aspects in their risk calculations that reflect personal and societal values, as well as affective responses. Both scientific experts and laypeople are subject to biases in their perceptions: People tend to judge themselves as less likely to suffer harm than others and see outcomes as more likely to happen if they are memorable, easy to imagine, or strongly affective.

At this point, we may ask, "How much risk is acceptable?" Evaluating acceptable risk depends on the desirability of the available options, and no definitive method is used for making the choice (Fischhoff, Lichtenstein, Slovic, Derby, & Keeney, 1981). "The *estimation* of risk is a scientific question—and therefore, a legitimate activity of scientists. . . . The *acceptability* of a given level of risk, however, is a political question, to be determined in the political arena" (Imperato & Mitchell, 1985, p. 26). At the individual level, acceptable risk is a personal decision: To fly or to take a train? To drink or not to drink? In Chapter 5, which addresses risk decisions, we will examine some of the ways in which individuals make choices about behaviors that carry potential risk.

Drinking has both risks and benefits, both of which are well known. Although studies of risk perception indicate that alcohol is viewed as having large risks and small benefits, such studies may reflect people's beliefs about alcohol problems as a societal issue, instead of about alcohol as a risky substance on a personal level. Consistent with a general optimistic bias, by which people perceive themselves as less vulnerable to risk than others, individuals view alcohol as an important general risk but a very small personal risk.

REFERENCES

Aas, H., Leigh, B. C., Anderssen, N., & Jakobsen, R. (1998). Two-year longitudinal study of alcohol expectancies and drinking among Norwegian adolescents. *Addiction, 93*, 373–384.

Agostinelli, G., & Miller, W. R. (1994). Drinking and thinking: How does personal drinking affect judgments of prevalence and risk? *Journal of Studies on Alcohol, 55*(3), 327–337.

Aitken, P. (1978). *Ten- to fourteen-year-olds and alcohol: A developmental study in the Central Region of Scotland.* Edinburgh: Her Majesty's Stationery Office.

Bennett, P. (1999). Understanding responses to risk: Some basic findings. In P. Bennett & K. Calman (Eds.), *Risk communication and public health* (pp. 3–19). Oxford, UK: Oxford University Press.

Bondy, S. J. (1996). Patterns of drinking and the acute consequences of alcohol use: Ontario, 1994. *Dissertation Abstracts International, 57*(4):2512-B.

Christiansen, B. A., Goldman, M. S., & Inn, A. (1982). Development of alcohol-related expectancies in adolescents: Separating pharmacological from social-learning influences. *Journal of Consulting and Clinical Psychology, 50*(3), 336–344.

Christiansen, B. A., Smith, G. T., Roehling, P. V., & Goldman, M. S. (1989). Using alcohol expectancies to predict adolescent drinking behavior after one year. *Journal of Consulting and Clinical Psychology, 57*(1), 93–99.

Critchlow, B. (1986). The powers of John Barleycorn: Beliefs about the effects of alcohol on social behavior. *American Psychologist, 41*(7), 751–764.

Finucane, M., Alhakami, A., Slovic, P., & Johnson, S. M. (2000). The affect heuristic in judgments of risks and benefits. *Journal of Behavioral Decision Making, 13*, 1–17.

Finucane, M. L., Slovic, P., & Mertz, C. K. (2000). Public perception of the risk of blood transfusion. *Transfusion, 40*(8), 1017–1022.

Fischhoff, B., Lichtenstein, S., Slovic, P., Derby, S. L., & Keeney, R. L. (1981). *Acceptable risk*. Cambridge, UK: Cambridge University Press.

Fischhoff, B., Slovic, P., & Lichtenstein, S. (1983). "The public" vs. "the experts": Perceived vs. actual disagreements about risks of nuclear power. In V. T. Covello, W. G. Flamm, J. V. Rodricks, & R. G. Tardiff (Eds.), *The analysis of actual versus perceived risks* (pp. 235–248). New York: Plenum.

Fisk, D. (1999). Perception of risk—Is the public probably right? In P. Bennett & K. Calman (Eds.), *Risk communication and public health* (pp. 133–139). Oxford, UK: Oxford University Press.

Freudenburg, W. R. (1988). Perceived risk, real risk: Social science and the art of probabilistic risk assessment. *Science, 242*(4875), 44–49.

Gigerenzer, G. (2000). *Adaptive thinking: Rationality in the real world*. New York: Oxford University Press.

Glassner, B. (1999). *The culture of fear: Why Americans are afraid of the wrong things*. New York: Basic Books.

Gustafson, R. (1988). Self-reported expected effects of a moderate dose of alcohol by college women. *Alcohol and Alcoholism, 23*(5), 409–414.

Gustafson, R. (1989). Self-reported expected emotional changes as a function of alcohol intoxication by alcoholic men and women. *Psychological Reports, 65*(1), 67–74.

Imperato, P. J., & Mitchell, G. (1985). *Acceptable risks*. New York: Viking.

Isaacs, M. (1977). Stereotyping by children of the effects of drinking on adults. *Journal of Studies on Alcohol, 38*(5), 913–921.

Jahoda, G., & Cramond, J. (1972). *Children and alcohol: A developmental study in Glasgow*. London: Her Majesty's Stationery Office.

Johnson, H. L., & Johnson, P. B. (1995). Children's alcohol-related cognitions: Positive versus negative alcohol effects. *Journal of Alcohol and Drug Education, 40*(2), 1–12.

Kasperson, R. E. (1992). The social amplification of risk: Progress in developing an integrative framework. In S. Krimsky & D. Golding (Eds.), *Social theories of risk* (pp. 153–178). Westport, CT: Praeger.

Keeney, R. L. (1994). Decisions about life-threatening risks. *New England Journal of Medicine, 331*(3), 193–196.

Lang, A., Murray, A., & Pelham, W. (1984). Children's perceptions of the effects of alcohol on adult-child interaction. Paper presented at the Annual Meeting of the Southeastern Psychological Association. New Orleans, LA.

Lang, A. R., Kaas, L., & Barnes, P. (1983). The beverage type stereotype: An unexplored determinant of the effects of alcohol consumption. *Bulletin of the Society of Psychologists in Addictive Behaviors, 2*(1), 46–49.

Lang, A. R., & Michalac, E. M. (1990). Expectancy effects in reinforcement from alcohol. In W. M. Cox (Ed.), *Why people drink: Parameters of alcohol as a reinforcer*. New York: Gardner Press.

Leigh, B. C. (1987). Beliefs about the effects of alcohol on self and others. *Journal of Studies on Alcohol, 48*(5), 467–475.

Leigh, B. C., & Stacy, A. W. (1994). Self-generated alcohol expectancies in four samples of drinkers. *Addiction Research, 1*, 335–348.

Lettieri, D. J., Sayers, M., & Pearson, H. W. (Eds.). (1980). *Theories on drug abuse: Selected contemporary perspectives* (NIDA Research Monograph No. 12). Washington, DC: U.S. Government Printing Office.

Lichtenstein, S., Slovic, P., Fischhoff, B., Layman, M., & Combs, B. (1978). Judged frequency of lethal events. *Journal of Experimental Psychology: Human Learning and Memory, 4*, 551–578.

Lindman, R., & Lang, A. R. (1986). Anticipated effects of alcohol consumption as a function of beverage type: A cross-cultural replication. *International Journal of Psychology, 21*(6), 671–678.

Lindman, R. E., & Lang, A. R. (1994). The alcohol-aggression stereotype: A cross-cultural comparison of beliefs. *International Journal of the Addictions, 29*(1), 1–13.

Lupton, D. (1999). *Risk.* London: Routledge.

Mäkelä, K., & Mustonen, H. (1988). Positive and negative experiences related to drinking as a function of annual alcohol intake. *British Journal of Addiction, 83*(4), 403–408.

Mäkelä, K., & Mustonen, H. (2000). Relationships of drinking behaviour, gender and age with reported negative and positive experiences related to drinking. *Addiction, 95*(5), 727–736.

Marín, G. (1996). Expectancies for drinking and excessive drinking among Mexican Americans and non-Hispanic Whites. *Addictive Behaviors, 21*(4), 491–507.

Marín, G., Posner, S.-F., & Kinyon, J.-B. (1993). Alcohol expectancies among Hispanics and non-Hispanic Whites: Role of drinking status and acculturation. *Hispanic Journal of Behavioral Sciences, 15*(3), 373–381.

Miller, P. M., Smith, G. T., & Goldman, M. S. (1990). Emergence of alcohol expectancies in childhood: A possible critical period. *Journal of Studies on Alcohol, 51*(4), 343–349.

Morgan, M. G. (1985). Powerline frequency electric and magnetic fields: A pilot study of risk perception. *Risk Analysis, 5*(2), 139–149.

Mustonen, H., & Mäkelä, K. (1999). Relationships between characteristics of drinking occasions and negative and positive experiences related to drinking. *Drug and Alcohol Dependence, 56*(1), 79–84.

National Research Council. (1996). *Understanding risk: Informing decisions in a democratic society.* Washington, DC: National Academy Press.

Nelkin, D. (1989). Communicating technological risk: The social construction of risk perception. *Annual Review of Public Health, 10*, 95–113.

O'Hare, T. (1995). Differences in Asian and White drinking: Consumption level, drinking contexts, and expectancies. *Addictive Behaviors, 20*(2), 261–266.

Paling, J., & Paling, S. (1994). *Up to your armpits in alligators? How to sort out what risks are worth worrying about.* Gainesville, FL: John Paling & Co.

Perloff, L. S., & Fetzer, B. K. (1986). Self-other judgments and perceived vulnerability to victimization. *Journal of Personality and Social Psychology, 50*(3), 502–510.

van der Pligt, J., Otten, W., & Richard, R. (1993). Perceived risk of AIDS: Unrealistic optimism and self-protective action. In J. B. Pryor & G. D. Reeder (Eds.), *The social psychology of HIV infection* (pp. 39–58). Hillsdale, NJ: Lawrence Erlbaum Associates.

Reese, F. L., & Friend, R. (1994). Alcohol expectancies and drinking practices among Black and White undergraduate males. *Journal of College Student Development, 35*(5), 319–323.

Rohsenow, D. J. (1983). Drinking habits and expectancies about alcohol's effects for self versus others. *Journal of Consulting and Clinical Psychology, 51*(5), 752–756.

Roizen, R. (1983). Loosening up: General population views of the effects of alcohol. In R. Room & G. Collins (Eds.), *Alcohol and disinhibition: Nature and meaning of the link* (Vol. NIAAA, Research Monograph No. 12, pp. 236–257). Washington, DC: U.S. Government Printing Office.

Ross, J. F. (1999). *Living dangerously: Navigating the risks of everyday life.* Cambridge, MA: Perseus Publishing.

Sjöberg, L. (1998). Risk perception of alcohol consumption. *Alcoholism: Clinical and Experimental Research, 22*(Suppl. 7), 277S–284S.

Skolbekken, J.-A. (1995). The risk epidemic in medical journals. *Social Science and Medicine, 40*(3), 291–305.

Slovic, P. (1987). Perception of risk. *Science, 236*(4799), 280–285.

Slovic, P. (1992). Perception of risk: Reflections on the psychometric paradigm. In S. Krimsky & D. Golding (Eds.), *Social theories of risk* (pp. 117–152). Westport, CT: Praeger.

Slovic, P. (1997). Risk perception and trust. In V. Molak (Ed.), *Fundamentals of risk analysis and risk management* (pp. 233–245). Boca Raton, FL: CRC Press.

Slovic, P. (1999). Trust, emotion, sex, politics, and science: Surveying the risk-assessment battlefield. *Risk Analysis, 19*(4), 689–701.

Slovic, P. (2000a). Do adolescent smokers know the risk? In P. Slovic (Ed.), *The perception of risk* (pp. 364–371). London: Earthscan Publications.

Slovic, P. (2000b). The perception and management of therapeutic risk. In P. Slovic (Ed.), *The perception of risk* (pp. 246–263). London: Earthscan Publications.

Slovic, P. (Ed.). (2000c). *The perception of risk.* London: Earthscan Publications.

Slovic, P., Finucane, M., Peters, E., & MacGregor, D. G. (2002). The affect heuristic. In T. Gilovich, D. Griffin, & D. Kahneman (Eds.), *Heuristics and biases: The psychology of intuitive judgment* (pp. 397–420). Cambridge, UK: Cambridge University Press.

Slovic, P., Finucane, M., Peters, E., & MacGregor, D. (in press). Risk as analysis and risk as feelings: Some thoughts about affect, reason, risk, and rationality. *Risk Analysis.*

Slovic, P., Fischhoff, B., & Lichtenstein, S. (1979). Rating the risks. *Environment, 21*(3), 14–20, 36–39.

Slovic, P., Fischhoff, B., & Lichtenstein, S. (1982). Facts versus fears: Understanding perceived risk. In D. Kahneman, P. Slovic, & A. Tversky (Eds.), *Judgment under uncertainty: Heuristics and biases* (pp. 463–489). Cambridge, UK: Cambridge University Press.

Slovic, P., Fischhoff, B., & Lichtenstein, S. (2000). Informing the public about the risks from ionizing radiation. In T. Connolly, H. R. Arkes, & K. R. Hammond (Eds.), *Judgment and decision making: An interdisciplinary reader* (pp. 114–126). Cambridge, UK: Cambridge University Press.

Spencer, J., & Crossen, C. (2003, April 24). Why do Americans feel that danger lurks everywhere? *Wall Street Journal,* A-1.

Spiegler, D. L. (1983). Children's attitudes toward alcohol. *Journal of Studies on Alcohol, 44,* 545–552.

Svenson, O., Fischhoff, B., & MacGregor, D. (1985). Perceived driving safety and seatbelt usage. *Accident Analysis and Prevention, 17*(2), 119–133.

Taylor, R. L. (1990). *Health fact, health fiction: Getting through the media maze.* Dallas, TX: Taylor Publishing Company.

Tversky, A., & Kahneman, D. (1974). Judgment under uncertainty: Heuristics and biases. *Science, 185,* 1124–1131.

Velez-Blasini, C. J. (1997). A cross-cultural comparison of alcohol expectancies in Puerto Rico and the United States. *Psychology of Addictive Behaviors, 11*(2), 124–141.

Weinstein, N. D. (1989). Perceptions of personal susceptibility to harm. In V. M. Mays, G. W. Albee, & S. F. Schneider (Eds.), *Primary prevention of AIDS* (pp. 142–167). Newbury Park, CA: Sage.

Zajonc, R. B. (1980). Feeling and thinking: Preferences need no inferences. *American Psychologist, 35,* 151–175.

Chapter 2

To Each His Own: Culture, Risk, and the Transgression of Boundaries

"Each culture is designed to use dangers as a bargaining weapon, but different types of cultures select different kinds of dangers for their self-maintaining purposes."

Mary Douglas, 1992

It is curious that in all societies, some risks are largely ignored while others elicit a strong response of anxiety and fear. Equally curious is the dual role often played by risk, as a positive attribute under some circumstances and a dangerous one under others. Where risk is seemingly encouraged in some areas of life, it is avoided in others.

It has been suggested that a preoccupation with risk occupies an inordinately prominent place in developed countries, reflecting their general affluence and the relative good health their citizens enjoy. Development, technology, and strides in medicine have faded the importance of many risks in the industrialized world, and their place has been taken by the increasing prominence of other risks brought about by shifting priorities in the nature and meaning of risk. Yet, in other parts of the world, where poverty, epidemics, and large-scale public health concerns prevail, risk assumes a different face. The ravages of HIV/AIDS, the threats of famine, war, drought, and floods, or simply the effort to stay alive from one day to the next are threats facing a large proportion of the world's population. The risk of living too close to power lines, the potential risk from eating food derived from genetically modified organisms, or the risks posed by certain types of tires or airbags in automobiles are not prominent sources of concern in situations where life's basic necessities must be met. This disparity in the saliency of certain risks also exists within individual societies, especially those in which the divide between rich and poor is wide.

It is unlikely, however, that economic disparities alone can account for the varied risks we face and the priority we might assign them. It is more likely that the roots of these disparities are found in the culture that defines different societies. Our view of the world around us is shaped largely by culture—the shared system of attitudes, goals, and practices, transcending language, and institutions that holds societies together. Culture is both a reflection of social cohesion and the cohesive force itself, determining and determined by shared values and beliefs. Culture establishes, to a large extent, the risks to which we will be exposed, what we consider risks, and how we prioritize and respond to these risks.

RISK AND THE COMPONENTS OF CULTURE

Let us begin by examining the components of culture that play a crucial role in the construction of risk. At the societal level, culture includes elements such as language, ideas, beliefs, customs, and institutions. It also comprises factors such as gender, age, ethnic heritage, and socioeconomic status that define the personal characteristics of those who live within a society. These factors bind together individuals, even if they do not share a common history or tradition or belong to the same societal strata. It should be emphasized that none of these variables exists in a vacuum, separate from the others. What ultimately shapes culture and the role it plays in the construction of risk is the interplay among these various factors, each significant in its own right, at the societal and individual level.

For many people, belonging to a particular demographic group based on gender, social position, or ethnicity is related to increased risk. It has been observed, for example, that in the U.S. suicide rates for Native American males between the ages of 25 and 34 is twice that of other ethnic groups. Alaskan Native males between the ages of 15 and 24 are 14 times more likely to commit suicide than young people in the U.S. in general (Substance Abuse and Mental Health Services Administration, 2002). Although the ethnicity of these individuals is not in itself a direct cause for heightened risk, it is accompanied by factors that are direct causes. Inadequate availability of health services, extreme poverty, geographic isolation, and culturally insensitive approaches to public health issues all contribute to the risk exposure of these groups. The same is true of other demographic factors that may not directly contribute to risk but, under certain cultural and social conditions, may be associated with heightened risk for some populations.

Gender

Biological differences between men and women, as well as gender roles in different cultures are important contributors to the risks people face. The saliency of certain risks varies for men and for women in general. In different parts of the world, risks may reach an even greater degree of variation (Murray & Lopez, 1996). Particularly in developing countries, the absence of adequate and readily available medical care represents a unique and often life-threatening risk for the populace. The risk is especially high for women because these factors contribute to the high rates of death during and as a result of childbirth. Other risks are also higher for women: They are more likely than men to be the victims of abuse and sex crimes and are more likely than men to live in poverty. The reasons often lie in the roles of women and in prevailing kinship roles in different societies, which make education, inheritance, and ownership of property difficult and contribute to economic deprivation, all of which lead to increased risk.

Men are also faced with their own sets of risks. Life expectancy for men is generally shorter than women in virtually all regions of the world. In particular, coronary heart disease is the major single cause of male mortality in most industrialized countries and, increasingly, in urban areas of developing countries (Murray & Lopez, 1996). Men are also more likely to die in traffic accidents and are at higher risk for a range of diseases, including cirrhosis of the liver, which is one of the 10 leading causes of male mortality.

The differences between the risk exposure of men and women are also, in part, due to gender differences in risk-taking behaviors and to their relative perceptions of risk, which are discussed at length in Chapter 1. Overall, men are greater risk takers than women, with younger men the most likely to engage in risky behaviors. Regarding the general perception of most risks, women tend to perceive risks as greater than do men (Flynn, Slovic, & Mertz, 1994). Sociological theories have offered a range of explanations for this behavioral pattern, including one that suggests that risk taking is closely related to survival, and that, from a theoretical standpoint at least, forgoing risks often means forgoing survival. Moreover, males are more likely to be presented with risky situations in which they are forced (or expected) to act to protect themselves and their families. They are more likely to be recruited into military service and be in professions such as law enforcement, in which a high degree of risk is present.

The Socioeconomic Divide

Socioeconomic status, often closely related to gender, has a significant impact on risk. Socioeconomic differences underlie more than only how people perceive risks. They also determine which risks are significant in our lives and their degree of saliency. Access to nutrition, health care, education, and a social network are directly related to risk exposure. The poor tend to be more vulnerable to risk and generally less able to cope adequately with its consequences. They are more at risk for injury, largely because of their environment, and have less access to health care. Violence and crime tend to affect the poor more than they do the rich, as do risks associated with old age and income insecurity or fluctuations in employment and the labor market.

The macro-level differential between those who are well-to-do and those who are poor is illustrated by the gap in life expectancies between developed and developing countries. According to the World Health Organization's Healthy Life Expectancy (World Health Organization [WHO], 2000) statistics, the highest average healthy life expectancy in the world is in Japan— 73.8 years. The lowest, in Sierra Leone, is only 29.5 years. Not surprising, the other 10 highest life expectancies can all be found in developed countries, while those at the bottom of the scale are found in sub-Saharan Africa. Over the last 10 years, the life expectancy in that region has dropped dramatically, largely due to the spread of AIDS. Similarly, infant mortality rates show a wide disparity— from a low of 3.53 deaths per 1,000 live births in Iceland to 144.38 deaths per 1,000 live births in Sierra Leone (U.S. Bureau of Census, 2003).

> Poverty means more than inadequate consumption, education, and health. As the voices of the poor cry out, it also means dreading the future—knowing that a crisis may descend at any time, not knowing whether one will cope. Living with such risk is part of life for poor people, and today's changes in trade, technology, and climate may well be increasing the riskiness of everyday life. Poor people are often among the most vulnerable in society because they are the most exposed to a wide array of risks (The World Bank, 2000).

Even in developed countries, such disparities are noticeable, especially with regard to health. In general, those with fewer economic advantages tend to be at greater risk for disease. This has been attributed to a number of factors, including psychosocial stress, poor diet, inadequate access to health care and tactics aimed at prevention of disease, and even genetic differences (Davey Smith, Gunnell, & Ben-Shlomo, 2001). A 1984 study of civil servants in the United Kingdom, known as the Whitehall study, showed that those in the lower echelons (e.g., clerical and manual) had a significantly higher risk than those in the upper echelons (administrative, professional, executive) (Marmot, Shipley, & Rose, 1984) both for mortality and for certain types of disease (Davey Smith, Shipley, & Rose, 1991).

The risk for mental illness and related problems also shows a strong relationship with poverty in both developed and developing countries. Research conducted in India, for instance, has focused on the relationship between poverty among subsistence farmers and the incidence of mental health problems. Depression and suicide rates among the socially and economically disadvantaged are particularly high (Patel, 2001). In the state of

Maharashtra, a disproportionate 82% of suicides were reported among the poorest segment of society, which constitutes only about 12% of that state's total population.

Curiously enough, poverty and deprivation are not the only factors that contribute to increased health risks. One phenomenon of today's developed societies is the emergence of health risks that are linked to the very lifestyles and conveniences that affluent societies have to offer. Over the past 25 years, obesity has increased dramatically across the population of the U.S. and is beginning to show similar trends in other industrialized nations. Given the strong association between obesity and a range of chronic medical conditions, health risks are on the rise. According to recent data, health care costs associated with obesity in the U.S. are currently almost twice those associated with smoking (Sturm, 2002).

Education

Education, closely linked to socioeconomic status, also relates to individual risk. It has been argued, for instance, that the lower exposure to many risks among those with higher levels of education (Sjöberg, 1998; Slovic, 1999) may be due, in part, to the level of understanding of particular risks that education offers, the resulting ability to do something about them, and the degree of control individuals feel they have over their lives. This is the principle underlying the notion of the "educated consumer," who is able to make an informed decision about the risks and potential levels of harm to which he or she will be exposed and over which there is a degree of control; however, education also relates directly to actual risk exposure. Those with knowledge and information can better understand the issues at hand and are thus able to reduce risk factors.

Age

In many ways, young people are exposed to a higher degree of risk than are adults. Infants and children, including adolescents, are still undergoing physical, intellectual, and emotional development, making them particularly vulnerable to a variety of factors. Many risks to which children are exposed are the result of socioeconomic factors, whether in developing or developed countries (Wadsworth, 1999). Malnutrition and infection are two of the major risks facing children early in life. Compounded by the lack of available health care, they account for the high infant mortality in many parts of the world. Socioeconomic adversity early in life appears to correlate with risk for mortality and disease in later years. Those in lower income groups tend to be exposed to a range of other risk factors, including smoking or high cholesterol (Faggiano, Partanen, Kogevinas, & Boffeta, 1997; Stronks, van de Mheen, Looman, & Mackenbach, 1997).

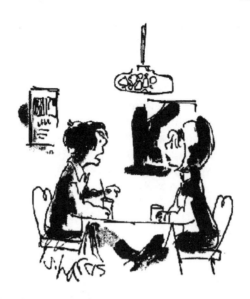

"MY BELIEF IS IF YOU'RE OLD ENOUGH TO
TAKE 'TEXTS, COUNTER-TEXTS AND META-TEXTS
IN WESTERN PHILOSOPHY', YOU SHOULD BE
OLD ENOUGH TO DRINK."

Because of their behavior, young people are generally more likely than adults to be exposed to risk. It appears that young people engage in risky behaviors partly because they simply ignore risks, perceive that risks are not likely to apply to them, or partly because of the satisfaction they expect to gain from such behaviors (Fromme, Katz, & Rivet, 1997). Thrill seeking is an attribute of youth, in which limits are tested and fate tempted. Young people generally believe that they will be able to control the consequences of their risk-taking behaviors (Slovic, 1999; Benthin et al., 1995; Plant & Plant, 1992). As a result, the numbers of young people at risk for injury and death from drunk driving accidents, unsafe sexual practices, experimentation with substance abuse, and other risky activities are high.

The relationship between age and risk does not apply exclusively to young people. The elderly, in general, are also at higher risk for a range of harms, primarily because of physical conditions and illness. No longer part of the workforce and without the security of a steady income, they are also at greater risk for poverty. Furthermore, with the disintegration of family structure in many places around the world, the elderly are at risk for dropping out of the social network, leaving them with little support and few resources. The often-precarious position of the elderly with respect to health and social issues also may color their perception of risk. In general, they are likely to be cautious and to perceive danger where it may or may not exist (Hennen & Knudten, 2001).

Ethnicity

One cannot discuss demographic variables without discussing the role ethnicity and cultural heritage play in defining risk. At the biological level, certain genetic components associated with race or a particular ethnic group may contribute significantly to risk. Whereas some of these components may increase risk, others may actually reduce it. For example, being at higher or lower risk for a genetic disorder is closely related to being part of a particular population group. At the biological level, a strong association exists among race, ethnicity, and certain genetic diseases. This relationship is very much a function of a history of endogamy rules (i.e., who can marry whom within certain group boundaries). For example, Ashkenazi Jews are at higher risk for Tay Sachs disease; individuals of West African descent are at greater risk for sickle-cell anemia; North Europeans at higher risk for cystic fibrosis; and individuals from the Mediterranean region at higher risk for beta-thalassemia (Burchard et al., 2003; Marteau & Richards, 1999).

Affiliation with a particular ethnic group is often regarded as an indicator, however crude, of socioeconomic disparity, particularly in multiracial and multiethnic societies. Rates of poverty among blacks and Hispanics (regardless of specific origin) in the U.S., for example, are three times higher than among whites as a group (National Center for Health Services, 1998). Similar profiles exist for other countries with heterogeneous populations. Thus, by virtue of this link with social status and conditions, the relationship between ethnicity and a range of health and social risks may be a close one.

It has been argued that the degree of power that can be exercised by certain groups over their own lives and the world around them relates closely to how they perceive risks. Being in control of one's own destiny is closely related to one's status within the social structure and the degree of perceived alienation from the social center. This phenomenon has been referred to as the "white male effect," based on the finding that white males generally tend to have the lowest perception of risk of any group studied (Flynn et al., 1994), interpreted as this demographic group's general position and social status. The "white male effect" may well reflect sociopolitical factors that determine acceptance and perceptions of risk and are linked in some societies to race or ethnicity. It is likely that disenfranchised groups may feel less in control of their fate because their exposure to risks may, in fact, be higher on balance. It is curious to note that advocates of risk acceptance generally tend to be white males.

Ample historical examples are available of how race and its relationship with social status are related to risk exposure. An extreme example of this relationship is the Tuskegee Syphilis Experiment, conducted between 1932 and 1972 by the U.S. Public Health Service. During this period, 399 poor, black male sharecroppers in Macon County, Alabama, were used as unwitting subjects to study the effects of late-stage syphilis. While telling their subjects that they were treating them for "bad blood," the physicians involved in the study ensured that those men did not receive any treatment for syphilis so that the progression of the disease could be observed unhindered (Jones, 1993). In the years since the study was exposed, it has achieved notoriety as a powerful symbol of the relationship between race, socioeconomic status, the structure of power, and actual exposure to risk.

NORMATIVE BEHAVIOR, BOUNDARIES, AND RISK

The interplay between demographic factors occupies an important place in risk construction, how we perceive risks, and the degree to which we are exposed to them. The relationship between demographics and risk is, to a large extent, also a reflection of social norms governing culture. Concepts of what is acceptable or normative behavior influence our perception of risk. Yet, what one culture defines as acceptable may be deemed unacceptable by another culture. Many familiar examples of potentially risky behaviors depend largely on views about risk held by a particular culture, including the use of seat belts in automobiles, engaging in extreme sports, or consuming certain foods. A certain degree of risk is clearly inherent in all of these behaviors; however, the way in which they are prioritized and whether they represent a considerable concern depends largely on cultural notions of what is acceptable, and, just as important, on views about the potential conse-quences of risky behavior.

It is striking for a visitor to the Netherlands, for example, to observe a large proportion of the population traveling by bicycle to work, to shop, and for enjoyment. According to statistics from the Dutch cities of Delft and Groningen, both of which boast extensive bikeway systems, at least 40% of trips in Delft and 50% of intracity journeys in Groningen are made by bicycle (ten Grotenhuis, 1986; Hartman, 1990; Huyink, 1987). If the visitor happens to be from the U.S., where cycling has largely been relegated to the realm of exercise, weekend entertainment, and leisure, perhaps an even more striking contrast is the absence of bicycle helmets among virtually all cyclists. The Netherlands is Europe's most densely populated country and has the most cars per square mile. Yet the Netherlands maintains more than 10,000 kilometers of bike paths and lanes—a ratio of 1:12 between cycle path and road miles—and cycling deaths per kilometer traveled are the lowest of any industrialized country studied (Preston, 1990).

This example illustrates how the same behavior may be adapted quite dif-ferently in different cultural environments. What is in one culture considered normal and commonplace may be regarded in another as highly risky, requiring protection, and outside the boundaries of everyday practice. The cultural perception of risk in either case may not make the actual act of cycling any more or less dangerous, but it does frame it within rather different contexts and allows different safeguards to be put into place. Perceived riskiness of certain behaviors is also shaped by the social stigma that may be associated with them. What is perceived as permissible behavior determines what lies outside the limits and thus should be marginalized and stigmatized. The line between the two is, in large part, culturally determined.

Exceptions exist, however. Many risks that ordinarily are avoided become desirable behaviors when undertaken for the greater good. Firefighters, police officers, and soldiers who consciously take risks that cross boundaries are exempt from the same rules and frameworks of risk that might apply in everyday life.

Explanations of how the concept of risk is constructed include the so-called culture theory (Douglas, 1992; Douglas & Wildavsky, 1982). According to this school of thought, risk is socially constructed and involves culturally learned assumptions and values: What people fear and how they fear it varies according to cultural concerns. In other words, according to social psychologist Paul Slovic (1999), hazards are real, but risk is socially constructed. The assessment of risk, therefore, is inherently subjective and represents a blending of science and judgment with important psychological, social, cultural, and political factors. The interplay among these elements may help to explain the dichotomy between desirable and undesirable risks.

As explained by culture theory, many people choose to engage in "risky" behavior after having weighed it within their particular cultural contexts. Decisions about risk are based on expectations and responsibilities accepted within that culture. Thus, when faced with risks, individuals make their judgments based on culturally learned assumptions and weightings. Risk is determined by accepted social boundaries. Or, to put it another way, risk is a mechanism for achieving social order. Boundaries, classifications, and taboos are set up to protect cultures from what threatens to destabilize them. All that falls outside these boundaries is generally regarded as threatening or "risky." Thus, in a sense, a potential risk represents a culture's response to the possible transgression of boundaries.

Consider the following example. Among bodybuilders, the use of steroids and analog drugs is widespread and serves to create group identity and maintain image. It is normal and expected behavior (Monaghan, Bloor, Dobash, & Dobash, 2000). Members of this group see themselves as distinct from the "junkies" who use the same drugs within a very different social context. This distinction allows not only for self-identification among bodybuilders as a group, but permits them to remove themselves from the stigma associated with drugs. In the view of this culture, the boundary for risk is not crossed by the "sensible" (i.e., athletic) user; transgressions by junkies into recreational use of these drugs represent risky behavior, possibly because of the link with behavioral loss of control. It is interesting that even though controlled drug use is acceptable and normative behavior within the body-builder subculture, use by women bodybuilders is regarded as "dangerous" and "polluting." Within this particular culture, the boundary is heavily guarded with respect to gender.

Normative behavior also reflects the influence of other factors, such as religion, in setting the limits for what constitutes risk. Religion is a powerful cultural mediator for defining many kinds of norms and boundaries. Evidence has shown that how religious individuals are and how actively they participate in the activities of their religion are strong predictors for abstinence from various behaviors (e.g., drinking, smoking, drug use, and sexual practices). This is true for young people (Koopmans, Slutske, van Baal, & Boomsma, 1999) and adults alike (Midanik & Clark, 1994). Religious beliefs set the boundaries for normative behavior, which, in turn, delineate the boundaries for risk. It has been suggested that close association with religious affiliation, regardless of denomination, leaves little room for individual choice. Those who practice their faith are motivated by their religion's prescriptions and proscriptions about risk boundaries.

A Cultural View of Health

Similar to many others, views about risks that relate to health are also strongly influenced by a given culture. In many instances, illness and the interpretation of its signs and symptoms are largely determined by a culture's ability to explain what cannot easily be understood. Culture-specific folk aspects still permeate our thinking about what is healthful or harmful, despite the great advances in and availability of Western medical information and health care. To a greater or lesser degree, for most people, illness still falls within a spectrum ranging from the supernatural to the natural (Trotter, 1985, 1991). An extreme example is the "evil eye," which poses a serious risk to health and well-being in certain cultures by drawing out the "vital essences" of the person exposed to it (Trotter, 1991). Other cultural views about health risk include the familiar notion that the common cold is "caught" by exposure to drafts (Baer et al., 1999).

Cultures have widely disparate ranges of views on "wellness" and on risks. Whereas in one culture certain lifestyles are regarded as the norm, elsewhere they may be quite unacceptable. The young and affluent urban dweller is more likely to be highly conscious of the relationship between diet, exercise, and health. Today, this awareness cuts across national lines, a by-product of globalization and the exchange of health information. For populations who live in rural or remote areas, or for those who are outside the mainstream of society for whatever reason, views on health and risk may be quite different.

Behavioral patterns and risks for chronic disease were examined among a population of Native Americans living on reservations in Montana (Nelson, Moon, Holtzman, Smith, & Siegel, 1997). The group included both adolescents and adults. Even in adolescents, most of the risk factors studied—smoking, smokeless tobacco use, infrequent consumption of fresh foods such as fruit and vegetables, and physical inactivity—were already prevalent. Similar results were observed in studies of the Maori of New Zealand, who are at much greater risk than their non-Maori counterparts are for illness and premature death. Lifestyles and the cultural view of health are among the major contributors to this risk, particularly where smoking, obesity, alcohol use, and accidents are concerned (Sachdev, 1990). In addition to accepting certain behaviors that might be viewed elsewhere as risky or unhealthy, these groups are generally outside of the mainstream, socially and economically, which in itself represents a risk factor.

Lifestyle choices based on cultural definitions of health are also prevalent in other societies in which accompanying risks affect much of the mainstream population. The case of male life expectancy in Russia provides another interesting insight into the relationship between risk and cultural views on health. It has been noted that life expectancy for men in Russia is lower than in many other countries and much lower than in the rest of Europe. Although life expectancy is generally on the rise in Eastern Europe, this is not the case in Russia. World Health Organization (WHO, 2000) figures published in 2000 indicate that although female babies born in Russia can generally expect to live until the age of 66.4, the life expectancy for male babies is only 56.1 years. These figures also represent one of the widest gender gaps in the world.

Explanations for the poor prognosis for Russian men attribute much of the problem to cultural factors, especially lifestyle. Russian culture typically includes heavy smoking and drinking, as well as the social acceptability of drunkenness, lack of exercise, and the lack of regular contact with the medical profession. Whereas some studies have pointed to drinking as playing a major role in lower life expectancy, the similarities in mortality rates between drinkers and nondrinkers argue for greater involvement of other lifestyle variables (Deev et al., 1998).

During the Soviet era, these lifestyles were facilitated by the availability of inexpensive cigarettes and alcohol, poor diets, and environmental pollution. Further contributing to these lifestyles were values endemic to the society in general, which placed great emphasis on the state, making the needs and well-being of the individual of secondary importance (Cockerham, 2000). Overall, the parameters for an unhealthy lifestyle were set and aided by cultural norms.

It should be pointed out, however, that the health risks evident within this population are not due to culture alone. Additional factors have no doubt made an important and deadly contribution. High levels of stress, economic hardship, and social alienation have characterized Russia throughout its years of political and economic transition. These factors, permeating all segments of society and cutting across gender lines, are reflected in the health of the population, in its lifestyle choices, and in an increased risk for illness and alcohol dependence (Palosuo, 2000).

Culture, Risk, and Alcohol

Cultures differ greatly in their views on the appropriateness of using certain substances. Alcohol and tobacco are perhaps the best-known examples; they are fully accepted in some cultures and shunned in others. However, the use of marijuana, opium, and even caffeine is also culturally sanctioned. According to Heath (2001),

> . . . the nature of a drug (or substance) is in large part defined by its cultural context. What some consider innocent leaves or seeds are viewed by others as psychoactive agents; a mild and refreshing beverage to some may be viewed as a mind-altering depressant by others. What in one culture is viewed as a minor analgesic, helpful in one's senior years, can be denounced as potentially addictive or harmful to an especially susceptible segment of the population. Even in similar and closely related cultures, wine is viewed as a food in France and as an alcoholic beverage in the United States. Drugs that are innocuous when consumed in an explicitly medical context or as part of a sacred ritual may result in untoward behavior when consumed in a recreational or secular context (p. 480).

The degree to which a substance is regarded as a potential risk to health and social well-being bears a close relationship to the extent it is integrated into the fabric of society. For the indigenous peoples of the Andes region, for example, the chewing of coca leaves is a commonplace and familiar activity. The leaves are chewed to prevent sickness and, among the very poor, are a means of relieving the sensation of hunger or thirst. Although coca is consumed in some well-delineated cultural settings, it is also chewed anywhere and anytime and represents a dietary staple.

The shaping of views regarding the acceptability or riskiness of particular substances is also closely linked to the moral stigma that may be associated with certain behaviors. Research has indicated that the negative social connotations of smoking, for example, as well as the high priority of smoking on the risk scale, are more closely related to the moralization of smoking as a behavior than to concerns about its health implications (Rozin & Singh, 1999). Similar views govern the consumption of alcohol in many cultures.

Much has been written about the myriad beliefs and practices associated with drinking around the world (Fekjaer, 1993; Heath, 1995, 2001; MacAndrew & Edgerton, 1969; Marshall, 1979). Various attempts have been made to create a cultural typology of drinking that is closely related to notions of risk and harm. These cultural positions range from "abstinent cultures" that are negative and prohibitive toward alcohol, and in which alcohol consumption is considered risky (for body and soul alike) and to be avoided, to "over-permissive cultures" that accept not only drinking but also intoxicated behavior and drinking pathologies (Pittman, 1967). Others have offered alternative explanations. Mäkelä (1983) separates cultural views of drinking based on their emphasis on either of alcohol's two main properties—its nutritional and intoxicating elements:

> In Italy and France, nutritional use of alcohol is historically dominant, but the French have developed more tolerant attitudes towards the intoxicant side effects of wine. Among the Jews, the Scandinavians and the Camba alike, alcohol is an intoxicant, but these three cultures have developed alternative normative solutions to the regulation of the use of this intoxicant. The ortho-dox Jews have succeeded in isolating alcohol into a sacral corner, the Camba use it up to extreme drunkenness but only on clearly demarcated occasions, and the Scandinavians vacillate between Dionysian acceptance and ascetic condemnation of drunkenness (p. 27).

Whatever typology one chooses to apply, some cultures view alcohol as medicine, while others see it as poison. Alcohol may be considered a stimulant or a relaxant, an adjunct to work or a marker of leisure, a complement to food or a substitute for it, or a symbol of high social status in some cultures and low social status in others (Heath, 2001).

Culture dictates the acceptability and perceived riskiness not only of certain drinking patterns, but also the relative acceptability of certain beverages. In some cultures, a social stigma is associated with "hard liquor" (distilled spirits). In others, where such beverages are traditionally produced and consumed, spirits are regarded as no more or less acceptable or risky than wine or beer. In reality, it is indisputable that all three beverage types— wine, beer, and distilled spirits—contain ethanol in varying amounts, making the risk distinction on the basis of alcohol alone a difficult one to base on scientific evidence.

Cultural notions about beverages are also linked to the taste preferences that prevail in different cultures. How else can one account for the popularity of certain beverage types among one population and the distaste for them in others? The fruit distillates of central Europe, *slivovitz* and *palinka,* are popular within that region, but may not be as popular in other parts of the world. Single malt whiskey, delicious to some, is an acquired taste for others, as is the Russian *kvaas* (a sweet beer made from bread) or *kumis,* the fermented mare's milk popular with the nomads of Mongolia (Heath, 2000).

The medicinal properties of beverage alcohol feature strongly in the lore and beliefs of folk medicine and bear a close connection with the risk that is thought to accompany its consumption. Stout beers were believed to possess nutritional properties that conferred strength upon those who drank them, and it was thought they could be consumed in place of food. Until well into the 20th century, stout beer was recommended as fortification for nursing mothers. The name "porter," in fact, is derived from the popularity of these beverages among the porters of London, who earned their keep carrying packages and used the beverage for strength. Even today, many folk remedies include alcohol-containing beverages to relieve colds or settle the stomach.

Cultural values are also associated with the relative acceptability or perceived riskiness of certain beverages for men and women, as well as for members of different social classes. In many cultures, a woman sipping a glass of white wine is considered more socially acceptable than a woman with a glass of bourbon in her hand. The wine drinker is often perceived as more sophisticated and less at risk for intoxication and other consequences than someone who drinks distilled spirits—the "hard stuff." In Poland, a traditionally spirits-drinking country, beer is commonly perceived as less "alcoholic," and its consumption, even in large quantities, less likely to result in intoxication and harm. Here, cultural views are closely related to the perceived risk for harm and, hence, affect exposure.

Alcohol is a psychoactive substance. It has the potential to alter mood and affect behavior. Although responsible drinking patterns can bring enjoyment, enhance quality of life, and may even confer health benefits upon those who practice them, reckless drinking may bring with it risks for a range of harm, both to the health of the individual and to society as a whole.

Drinking Patterns and Health Risk

In the countries of the Mediterranean region, as well as in certain countries of Middle Europe, such as Hungary, the risks for the chronic harms of drinking, especially liver cirrhosis, are high (Corrao, 1998; Racz, Vingender, Schaffer, & Pakozdi, 1999). These risks have been linked to the prevailing drinking patterns, often characterized by chronic heavy drinking. In the countries of Northern Europe, on the other hand, more typical patterns involve heavy and episodic drinking, increasing the risk for acute harm—notably accidents and injuries. Although variations on this rather simplistic dichotomy certainly exist, the basic relationships hold true.

Whether alcohol consumption is viewed in the context of its outcomes for the individual or for society, drinking potentially carries risks that are by no means negligible. Yet, how such risks are perceived is closely related to cultural views on alcohol and the concept of "normal" drinking. It is this view of normative drinking behavior that delineates the perceived boundary for risk and the threshold at which this boundary is crossed. Across cultures, the range of drinking levels described as "normal" is broad. In Greece and Spain, for instance, there is generally little concern about the quantity of alcohol consumed with meals. In India and the U.S., on the other hand, where drinking and eating are not well-integrated activities, this may not be considered an acceptable concept of "normal" drinking.

The cultural positioning of drinking has also been correlated with the variation in rates of drinking problems across countries. It has been suggested, for example, that the complexity of the social and political organization of a society correlates negatively with drunkenness. Thus, a culture with a rigid and highly stratified social structure is likely to experience less drunkenness, perhaps due to its clearly defined social boundaries for acceptable and unacceptable drinking behaviors. In more egalitarian societies, such as the Scandinavian countries, one is likely to encounter more drunkenness (Room & Mäkelä, 2000). Even in preliterate societies, social control and social and political power relationships are important factors that influence drinking customs and levels of alcohol consumption.

It is important to point out, however, that risks associated with alcohol consumption are not related solely to heavy drinking patterns or the incidence of drunkenness. Many adverse outcomes of drinking, particularly acute problems such as accidents, have been attributed to the "normal" drinker. In fact, the Prevention Paradox (Kreitman, 1986) postulates that it is the normal drinker—who generally drinks moderately but occasionally drinks excessively or irresponsibly (e.g., driving while impaired)—who contributes to the majority of problems.

In addition to defining the role of alcohol in society and the related behaviors that may or may not be deemed "risky," culture also influences some of the more objective measures of risk, namely the symptoms that are considered indicators of risk for alcohol dependence (Schmidt & Room, 1999). Curiously, cultural definitions apply to both the more subjective psychological symptoms of dependence and to the objective physical ones. The threshold above which particular symptoms are recognized as serious varies significantly, as does whether such symptoms even are considered as alcohol problems or should simply be accepted as part and parcel of drinking.

One criterion for diagnosing alcohol dependence, for example, is the requirement for a "period of heavy drinking." How long such a period lasts appears to be open to interpretation; an important cultural difference exists in the distinction between a 2-week and a 4-week period in terms of diagnosis among certain groups. Whereas most Native American tribes are generally abstinent and others are moderate drinkers, groups with a "well-defined cultural pattern of binge or episodic heavy drinking" also exist. Results of cross-cultural studies found that for these groups, the 2-week period of drinking would generally not be viewed as problematic, while the longer period of 4 weeks would. Such conceptual differences also exist in other cultures with regard to thresholds at which criteria and diagnoses would be applicable. A behavior considered normal and not significant from a medical point of view in one culture may be regarded as diagnostic in another.

In some cultures, symptoms of alcohol abuse or dependence are considered relatively benign or even positive. For example, drunkenness may be considered socially acceptable, even as "heroic" drinking, by which the drinker demonstrates resilience and strength in relation to alcohol. In others, notably those with a tradition of temperance, experiences associated with drinking may be considered problematic at a much lower threshold.

A particular culture's views on risk are reflected in its responses to them. In the case of alcohol, significant variation exists in the degree to which problem drinkers are stigmatized in society, how legislation is enacted and enforced, and how penalties are meted out. Approaches to prevention and treatment also resonate differently with different groups. The treatment field has long been engaged in a debate regarding the relative effectiveness of complete abstinence or controlled drinking (which may even allow for a return to moderate drinking) for alcohol-dependent individuals and for minimizing future risk to self and others. The relative acceptance of different approaches is strongly dependent upon culture.

One need not look to the extremes of alcohol consumption to find examples of cultural variation in the perception of associated risk. Cultural acceptability of drinking by pregnant women offers an excellent example of the relationship between alcohol, culture, and demographics. In a number of countries around the world, official guidelines for alcohol consumption proscribe drinking by pregnant women (International Center for Alcohol Policies [ICAP], 1999). Several reasons for this exist, but the recommendations are motivated primarily by a concern for the effects on the health of the unborn child and, in particular, the risk for serious developmental deficits such as fetal alcohol syndrome (FAS) or fetal alcohol effects (FAE). The risk for FAS is quite high in certain areas of the world, notably the Western Cape region of South Africa (Croxford & Viljoen, 1999; Viljoen, 1999; May et al., 2000). A high prevalence has also been documented among particular subpopulations, such as subgroups of Native American women who are heavy drinkers (Fleming & Manson, 1990; Ma, Toubbeh, Cline, & Chisholm, 2002). Globally, however, FAS is relatively uncommon (Abel, 1995).

Even though the exact drinking level at which the risk for FAS is heightened has not been established, it is clear from the scientific evidence that it is associated almost exclusively with high and chronic levels of alcohol consumption, usually among problem drinkers (Abel, 1999; O'Leary, 2002; Plant, Abel, & Guerri, 1999; Royal College of Obstetricians and Gynaecologists [RCOG], 1999). No clear evidence exists to prove that women who consume an occasional drink during pregnancy, or even those who drink at low or moderate levels, are likely to experience any adverse effects to themselves or their children, although no definitively "safe" level has been established.

Yet, the perception that any amount of alcohol consumption during pregnancy does pose a serious risk has become part of the cultural attitude toward drinking in some parts of the world. In the U.S., drinking by pregnant women is generally frowned upon; this is an attitude curiously at odds with the recommendation from another highly industrialized country, the United Kingdom. RCOG, while cautious, does not advise against one drink a day (RCOG, 1999). Similar advice is given by the Australian government in its newly released official drinking guidelines (National Health & Medical Research Council, 2001). Clearly, although some degree of risk is real, culture plays an important role in societal views on alcohol and pregnancy and in views of drinking by women in general.

Drinking Patterns and Risk to Society

The interpretation and perception of risks that certain patterns of alcohol consumption may pose to society are also determined, in large part, by culture. Although accidents and public disorder resulting from reckless drinking present a challenge to society and involve significant social cost, they may not be viewed in the same light in every culture.

Perceptions of risk inherent in drinking and driving, its social acceptability, and the enforcement of laws that attempt to minimize accidents are an interesting example of the role culture can play in determining the societal risks posed by drinking. A comparative study of attitudes on drinking and driving in Italy, the U.S., and Norway suggests significant cultural differences (Flaminio, 1989; Poldrugo & Flaminio, 1990). The study showed that individuals in the U.S. are more likely to drink and drive, even after consuming large quantities of alcohol, than are individuals in either Italy or Norway.

Research conducted within the U.S., a multiethnic society, also supports the notion that different cultural groups—Caucasian, Hispanic, Asian—have diverging views on drinking and driving. They may have varying perceptions on the permissible threshold for drinking, the effects of alcohol, and whether driving while intoxicated is acceptable behavior. Often, members of these groups have differing levels of knowledge and awareness of the laws that govern drinking and driving and the penalties for offenders (Cherpitel & Tam, 2000; Royal, 2000a, 2000b).

These results are not surprising given the cultural differences in the acceptance of norms around drinking and "drinking culture." British consumers, for instance, are reportedly highly likely to underestimate the potency of their drinks. In addition, the prevailing pub culture, which encourages Britons to do much of their drinking outside the home, contributes both to the likelihood of traffic accidents and to the perception of drinking and driving as less risky (Snortum, 1990).

Demographic variables also relate to how risks around drinking and driving are constructed. Younger individuals—particularly young males, who make up a large proportion of traffic fatalities in many countries—are typically more prone to thrill seeking than their elders and more likely to discount the risks associated with drinking and driving. As some of the examples of differences in perception among ethnic and national groups have shown, education about legislation and the effects of alcohol also plays an important role in how the risks associated with drinking and driving are perceived.

Drunkenness

Public disorder and drunkenness are societal risks closely related to certain drinking patterns and to perceptions and cultural views of risk. Drunkenness and disorderly behavior that can result from it are largely defined by a culture's boundaries for normative and acceptable behavior. Such behavior is often the reflection of particular social dynamics and may have culturally symbolic value. The concept of drunkenness is very much defined by where "sober" ends and "drunk" begins, and by the expectation of what constitutes drunken behavior and what is permissible under different circumstances.

It also depends on what is regarded as acceptable "second-hand" risk associated with drunkenness—risk not to the drinker but to those around him or her. For example, the impact of drunken behavior of college students on their friends and roommates has been described (Wechsler, Lee, Nelson, & Lee, 2001). Families, spouses, and children also experience the second-hand effects of drunkenness in the form of drained economic resources, absence, disruption of family life, and, in some cases, violent behavior. The extent to which such exposure is tolerated and considered acceptable or risky varies among cultures.

In most cultures, drunkenness, especially public drunkenness, is generally not condoned and represents a public order and public health concern. In certain cultures, however, drunken behavior is tolerated (or even encouraged) as long as it is confined to well-defined contexts and occasions. The parameters for these conditions are largely shaped by the prevailing attitudes toward drinking in general and by a society's definition of what constitutes permissible behavior associated with drinking (MacAndrew & Edgerton, 1969). These attitudes are inextricably linked with the disinhibitive properties of alcohol and are shaped by the prevailing views on the appropriateness of disinhibition and the potential risk it may represent. Whereas "letting one's hair down" may be acceptable among some groups, others do not sanction it.

Some societies use drunkenness to separate groups from each other and to mark class distinctions. While being drunk may be permissible for some members of society, often males and those higher in the social hierarchy, it may be forbidden to others. Within this context, the consumption of alcohol (or abstention from drinking in some cultural contexts), as well as the right to become drunk, are used in a symbolic sense to achieve cohesiveness within groups while setting them apart from others. Drunkenness also reflects the notions of risk as they apply to different groups. Although competitive drinking may be encouraged among men, a tipsy or drunken woman is generally considered unsavory. The potential risks involved in being drunk are generally perceived to be higher for women than for men.

Yet, some cultures permit "time-outs," which are temporary suspensions of both cultural sanctions against drunkenness and the accompanying notions about risk. Such time-outs usually occur during festivals and celebrations, but, again, only in a well-defined context. These occasions are frequently the exclusive domain of men and aimed at heightening group identity (although the no-holds-barred merriment during Mardi Gras is a notable exception).

Whereas public drunkenness on regular occasions might be forbidden and even punishable, it may be expected behavior during time-outs, including, for example, its role in ritual symbolism. In many societies, ritualized intoxication is integrated into drinking behavior. Among the Aztecs, inebriation was expected on holy days, but public drunkenness on secular occasions was forbidden and punished with penalties ranging from public disgrace to death by stoning or beating (Madsen & Madsen, 1979). Only the aged were exempt from social sanctions prohibiting public drunkenness.

TIME SHIFTS AND TRENDS

Culture is not static; instead, it is fluid and constantly evolving. Languages change over time, political and social conditions ebb and flow, and population-level demographics shift. Such transformations are accompanied by changes in definitions of social boundaries, as well as by changes in the construction of risk.

Much of the transformation in the immediacy of risks is, for better or worse, attributable to globalization. Both the perception of risk and the actual risks themselves have diminished for many people in the modern world. Overall, we are likely to lead longer and healthier lives, have greater access to medical care, better nutrition, and more educational opportunities that offer an improved quality of life. Although these positive trends are clearly more likely to occur in developed and affluent societies, many of them can be felt even in developing countries. These changes have, in large part, accompanied globalization and the greater ease and efficiency in communication and the sharing of resources.

Despite such encouraging trends, the face of risk around the world has grown more terrifying at the same time. Certain threats, once localized, now represent risks for greater numbers of people in an increasing number of places. The threat of bioterrorism has become a reality. Global military involvement in regional conflicts can easily expand these clashes beyond their immediate boundaries.

Greater interconnectedness between people has been both a blessing and a menace to society. Although it allows greater ease in communication and greater access to the benefits of modern life, it also means that certain risks, often previously confined to remote areas of the world, can spread at a dizzying pace. Diseases like Sudden Acute Respiratory Syndrome (SARS) can now spread between continents in a matter of hours, making their containment difficult and their proliferation unpredictable.

Although risks and the saliency we attribute to them may be changing more quickly than ever in today's fast-paced world, shifting trends centering on cultural boundaries, behaviors, and risk perception are not a novel phenomenon. Cultures are continuously evolving for historical, social, or economic reasons, and this evolution bears directly on the understanding of risk and harm. As the relative status of risks has changed, so have corresponding societal responses.

Each age has had its share of risk in its list of priorities. Even within the same culture, the fluid nature of how risks are perceived and addressed over time may undergo significant transformation. As societal boundaries around behaviors and acceptability are redrawn repeatedly, what may fall well within the norm at one point in time may be well outside its limits at another time. The relationship between American society and alcohol offers a dramatic illustration of cultural ebb and flow and the changing role of risk.

From Godly Creature to Demon Rum

By all accounts, America in the 1800s was fast becoming a nation of drunkards. During the first three decades of the 19th century, the average American—man, woman, and child—consumed larger amounts of alcohol per year than at any other point during the nation's history (Rorabaugh, 1979). It is estimated that between 1800 and 1830, the annual per capita consumption in the U.S. peaked at levels approximating 19 liters of pure alcohol. By comparison, in 2001, annual per capita consumption was roughly 7 liters (World Advertising Research Center [WARC], 2003). From the vantage point of the 21st century, when some 40% of the U.S. population consists of abstainers (ICAP, 2000) and proscriptions against drinking and laws regulating the availability of alcohol are more rigid than those in many other countries, these figures are more than a little surprising.

The culture surrounding alcohol in American society and the perception of risks associated with its consumption clearly underwent a significant shift over the course of two centuries. It is curious to consider the characterization of 19th-century Americans as "certainly not as sober as the French or Germans, but perhaps about on a level with the Irish" (Rorabaugh, 1979). Today, Ireland has the 3rd highest level of per capita consumption in the world. France and Germany follow in 6th and 8th place, respectively, while the U.S. is 26th on the list (WARC, 2003).

Not only were the levels at which Americans drank dramatically different from what they are today, so were their drinking patterns. Drinking accompanied most daily activities and routines. The mid-morning foray to the tavern represented the equivalent of today's coffee break, and the most popular beverages of choice were by far distilled spirits—whiskey, rum, gin, and brandy. Alcohol was generally accepted as part of American life among all social and occupational groups. Even in the strongholds of temperance, such as the country's seminaries, students regularly consumed brandy toddies. According to the Reverend Increase Mather, alcohol should be regarded as a "creature of God."

Nineteenth-century attitudes about drinking and children provide perhaps the most striking example of the change that alcohol has undergone in American society. They illustrate the extent to which the boundaries and risks associated with drinking have been redrawn. White males (for alcohol was largely prohibited for the mostly enslaved blacks of the day) were taught to drink from their early childhood. Rorabaugh (1979) writes, "(a)s soon as a toddler was old enough to drink from a cup, he was coaxed to consume the sugary residue at the bottom of an adult's nearly empty glass of spirits. Many parents intended this early exposure to alcohol to accustom their offspring to the taste of liquor, to encourage them to accept the idea of drinking small amounts, and thus to protect them from becoming drunkards" (Rorabaugh, p. 14). This approach to alcohol education is certainly a far cry from the drinking age of 21 in effect in the U.S. today, which is the highest in the world (ICAP, 1998).

The 1830s witnessed a dramatic drop in alcohol consumption and a cultural shift from a heartily drinking nation to one where zealous abstainers gained momentum. Many reasons exist for the shifting viewpoint of alcohol as a blessing and one of life's pleasures to its status as Demon Rum, a destroyer of households and a portal to poverty, violence, and despair. It has been argued that the rise of temperance was but one of the many reform movements that took place in 19th-century American society. Others have interpreted this shift as a reaction on the part of the clergy and the middle class to the threat posed to their social status by the rise of powerful industrialists. The temperance movement, however, was also undoubtedly a response to the prevailing drinking patterns of the times, particularly the excesses and binges that brought harm to individuals and society alike.

The result of this cultural about-face was that by 1855, legal prohibition had been adopted in 13 of 40 states and territories. Temperance societies were on the rise, and their platforms for reform were often much broader than merely a focus on alcohol. The Women's Christian Temperance Union, for example, pushed for equal legal rights for women, as well as for the right to vote, the institution of kindergarten, and an attack on the smoking of tobacco (Musto, 1996). The antialcohol movement in the U.S. culminated in Prohibition, lasting almost 14 years. Even after the repeal of Prohibition, drinking remained, and still remains, poorly integrated into the fabric of everyday life. The prevailing attitudes surrounding alcohol in the U.S. are influenced predominantly by a focus on risk and the need to treat alcohol with caution.

Neckties and Coca-Cola®

One of the main impacts of globalization has been on the identity and integrity of individual cultures, as well as their values and norms. In many parts of the world, traditional lifestyles have undergone significant upheaval. There has been much criticism that these changes are encouraging an influx of "Western" values into societies that are not ready to absorb them, leaving societal norms at odds with some of the novel ways of life that are being introduced. There is concern that the clash of cultures is breaking down barriers that have traditionally served to maintain integrity and order, and that, as a result, a new generation of risks has been created.

These changes are visible both at the societal level, manifested in large-scale cultural shifts, and the individual level, as mobility from one part of the world to another becomes more routine. Societies that previously were demographically static are becoming increasingly heterogeneous with the influx of immigrants and expatriates. The resulting melding of cultures demands that new values and lifestyles be incorporated into existing ones.

Such demographic integration has also changed the way certain risks are perceived. The rise of anti-immigrant sentiments in a number of European countries, for example, appears within this context to be an expression of risk perception. The unfamiliarity of individuals who look different, speak a different language, and bring with them new lifestyles and traditions represents risk in the minds of many. Resistance to these changes represents an attempt to reinforce traditional cultural boundaries and preserve the integrity of the existing social order.

There is evidence that risks have also taken on new meaning and prominence in the area of health. A close relationship appears to exist between today's hurried pace of life and resulting unhealthy lifestyles, giving rise to so-called "modern health worries" (Petrie et al., 2001) that create a new family of health risks, which include environmental pollution, toxins, tainted foods, and radiation. Where such worries play a prominent role, adverse health effects have been observed: a higher incidence of intolerance to foods as well as conditions such as chronic fatigue syndrome, one of the more perplexing illnesses of our time. Some of these health risks have been directly linked to environmental factors, such as multiple chemical sensitivity, immune system dysfunction, electric allergy, total allergy syndrome, and "20th-century disease," although conclusive explanations have not been found to date (Petrie et al., 2001).

Although it is possible that these new illnesses do indeed emanate from our changing environment and our "modern" way of life, an alternative explanation is that we may increasingly be attributing certain common health problems and other physical complaints to environmental factors. It may well be, after all, that having eliminated many of the risks they once faced, modern, affluent societies are now engaging in problem inflation and creating new risks to occupy those that have been conquered.

Shifting Risks and Drinking

Neither drinking patterns nor the perceptions of risks associated with them have been exempt from change. This is well illustrated by the rise and fall in popularity of certain beverages that are, at times, the height of fashion and, at others, poison to be banned and shunned. Perhaps the most praised and equally the most reviled of these has been *absinthe*, the "green fairy," or *fée verte*, which once inspired the likes of Verlaine, Rimbaud, Baudelaire, van Gogh, Hemingway, and Wilde.

La fée verte (La Fée Verte Absinthe House, 2003)

After the first glass you see things as you wish they were. After the second you see things as they are not. Finally, you see things as they really are, and that is the most horrible thing in the world.

Oscar Wilde

There is not a regimental surgeon who will not tell you that absinthe has killed more Frenchmen in Africa than the flittá, the yataghan, and the guns of the Arabs put together.

Alexandre Dumas

The man let the water trickle gently into his glass, and as the green clouded, a mist fell from his mind.

Ernest Dowson, Absinthe Taetra

Our awareness of the risks associated with certain patterns of drinking has increased dramatically over the last several decades. In many ways, it is not just awareness that has increased but the risks themselves, which are, in fact, greater today than before. Our increased reliance on motor vehicles, for instance, does not mix well with certain drinking behaviors. There is greater awareness of the social and medical implications of drinking and a greater perceived need to address and prevent possible harm. As a result, there have been changes in how risks associated with drinking are defined.

Like most other things, drinking cultures are not static and patterns evolve over time, responding to social, political, and economic changes. This is true for virtually every drinking culture around the world, although in some cultures the change is more marked than in others. In many cultures, the traditional role of alcohol is gradually being displaced. The countries of the Mediterranean region, where alcohol consumption was traditionally considered an adjunct to meals, are experiencing a shift in drinking patterns. It has been reported that young people are now drinking "American style," and among the general population, traditional beverages are being displaced. In France and Spain, long known as wine-drinking countries, there has been a significant decrease in wine consumption over the past two decades, while the consumption of beer, previously not a popular beverage, has increased (WARC, 2003).

Many cultures have traditionally reserved a special place for alcohol around symbolic occasions and celebrations (Heath, 2000). This allowed them to maintain social boundaries for risk with respect to alcohol. Yet, many of these traditions are changing, and alcohol is increasingly consumed outside of special occasions. In Poland, for instance, alcohol was traditionally consumed primarily on holidays and at ceremonies, generally in large quantities but on infrequent occasions. Drinking was closely linked with camaraderie, and solitary drinking was viewed as generally unacceptable (Zielinski, 1994). The fall of the Soviet Bloc and the opening of Poland to the West brought with it changes in lifestyle that impact the traditional culture. As a result, the "party" or the practice of dropping by for a drink with friends has become increasingly popular, particularly among the educated classes in urban areas. The drinking of large quantities of alcohol has similarly moved to more frequent and less "special" occasions, bringing with it a new set of risks.

The "Westernization" of Polish drinking patterns has also caused a shift in the beverages consumed by various segments of the population. Traditionally a spirits-drinking culture, where vodka was considered the beverage of choice, in recent years, Poland has seen an increase in the popularity of beer, which currently represents an estimated 50% of the beverage alcohol consumed. Because of the cultural view that only spirits constitute "real" alcohol, beer is not regarded as an alcohol-containing beverage, a perception that has considerable impact on drinking patterns and the risks for harm associated with them.

Not all shifts in relation to alcohol consumption have been in the direction of increased risk for harm. Indeed, the perception of and, consequently, the exposure to many risks have undergone favorable changes as certain behaviors have become less acceptable. For example, awareness of the risks associated with drinking and driving has increased in many places, as has the social stigma associated with it. Much of this shift has come about through greater public awareness of the impairing effects of drinking on driving ability and reaction time. Resulting social pressure and legal enforcement are gradually bringing about a change in behavior. Designated drivers are not uncommon in many cultural contexts, and harm reduction measures, such as the training of serving staff in drinking establishments, reflect a positive development.

Although trends and shifts in culture are clearly visible in the developed world, in developing countries they are perhaps even more prominent, particularly where traditional lifestyles and cultural norms are greatly at odds with the influences of globalization. Living conditions have changed dramatically in many of these countries, often widening the gap between the "haves" and the "have-nots." Many developing countries are regarded as emerging markets for the goods and lifestyles developed countries have to offer, further accelerating this process. As a result, a backlash has occurred against such outside influences in many parts of the world, representing an attempt to safeguard culture by maintaining social structure, boundaries, and roles.

Traditional drinking patterns and the role of alcohol in society have shifted radically in many developing countries, also changing the face of risk. Perhaps the most poignant example of such change is the introduction of alcohol into cultures in which it was previously unknown or rarely consumed, such as to the Basarwa people (or Bushmen) of southern Africa.

Alcohol-containing beverages are not featured in traditional Basarwa culture, and moderate drinking is virtually unknown, although some alcohol was traditionally consumed in a mild form and within certain well-defined social boundaries for the promotion of social cohesion and for ritual purposes (Macdonald & Molamu, 1999). After Botswana gained its independence in 1966, restrictions on alcohol availability dating back to colonial times were lifted and a range of beverages flooded the market. Around the same time, however, dramatic changes were also taking place in the lifestyles of the Basarwa, who increasingly moved to the squalor of semiurban squatting environments. Cheap, low quality, home-produced beverage alcohol is easily accessible and readily consumed by a group of people who are generally disenfranchised and without much hope for the future. Alcohol problems among the Basarwa reportedly have reached epidemic proportions. The Basarwa's traditional and well-delineated drinking culture was disrupted by the cultural shifts that occurred within their environment.

Another well-known historical example is offered by the introduction of beverage alcohol among the indigenous peoples of North America. Although various psychoactive substances were known and widely used by some tribes (again, within well-defined boundaries and occasions), alcohol was not. As a result, the relationship some tribes have since developed with alcohol has been a difficult one, fraught with risk, and resulting in large part from the lack of a supportive social framework. Similarly, the Aboriginal people of Australia have been left to deal with the risks created by the introduction of alcohol into their traditional culture. Like the Basarwa and Native American peoples, they are largely outside the mainstream of society, and, among them, not only is heavy drinking widespread, but also the abuse of a range of substances, including alcohol, tobacco, marijuana, amphetamines, cocaine, heroin, and inhalants (Gracey, 1998; Gray & Chickritz, 2000).

SUMMARY

How risks are perceived and the degrees to which individuals and groups are exposed to them are shaped by culture on a variety of levels. The variables of culture and demographics, including age, gender, and socioeconomic status, help to shape notions about risk while simultaneously shaping the very risks to which individuals are exposed.

Risk, however, is also a mechanism for maintaining boundaries, minimizing harm, and dealing with the unfamiliar and the dangerous at both individual and societal levels. Definitions of risk are shaped in large part by what cultures define as normative behavior and by what they deem acceptable. In this sense, the notion of risk is useful in maintaining the status quo.

When dealing with risk, it is important to remember that cultural definitions of boundaries and normative behavior differ significantly, and that the prioritization and saliency of risks vary a great deal in different parts of the world. When interpreting risks and attempting to address them at the level of intervention or policy, it is therefore essential to bear these cultural differences in mind. Only when risks are viewed, to the extent possible, within their cultural context and against the backdrop of what is acceptable, appropriate, and normative behavior, can we hope to begin to understand them.

In the next chapter, we examine the issue of how potentially risky situations are communicated to the public, how the source of such information affects the message, and how discrepancies and misconceptions about the degree of risk involved can occur in the process.

REFERENCES

Abel, E. L. (1995). An update on incidence of FAS: FAS is not an equal opportunity birth defect. *Neurotoxicology and Teratology, 17,* 437–443.

Abel, E. L. (1999). What really causes FAS? *Teratology, 59,* 4–6.

Baer, R. D., Weller, S. C. P. L., Trotter, R., Garcia de Alca Garcia, J., Glazer, M., Klein, R., et al. (1999). Cross-cultural perspectives on the common cold: Data from five populations. *Human Organization, 58,* 251–260.

Benthin, A., Slovic, P., Morgan, P., Severson, H., Mertz, C. K., & Gerrard, M. (1995). Adolescent health-threatening and health-enhancing behaviors: A study of word association and imagery. *Journal of Adolescent Health, 17,* 143–152.

Burchard, E. G., Ziv, E., Coyle, N., Gomez, S. L., Tang, H., Karter, A. J., et al. (2003). The importance of race and ethnic background in biomedical research and clinical practice. *New England Journal of Medicine, 348,* 1170–1175.

Cherpitel, C. J., & Tam, T. W. (2000). Variables associated with DUI offender status among Whites and Mexican Americans. *Journal of Studies on Alcohol, 61,* 698–703.

Cockerham, W. C. (2000). Health lifestyles in Russia. *Social Science & Medicine, 51,* 1313–1324.

Corrao, G. (1998). Liver cirrhosis mortality trends in Eastern Europe, 1970–1989: Analyses of age, period and cohort effects and of latency with alcohol consumption. *Addiction Biology, 3,* 413–422.

Croxford, J., & Viljoen, D. L. (1999). Alcohol consumption by pregnant women in the Western Cape. *South African Medical Journal, 89,* 962–965.

Davey Smith, G., Gunnell, D., & Ben-Shlomo, Y. (2001). Life-course approaches to socio-economic differentials in cause-specific adult mortality. In D. Leon & G. Walt (Eds.), *Poverty, inequality and health: An international perspective* (pp. 88–124). Oxford, UK: Oxford University Press.

Davey Smith, G., Shipley, M. J., & Rose, G. (1991). Socioeconomic differentials in cancer among men. *International Journal of Epidemiology, 20,* 339–345.

Deev, A., Shestov, D., Abernathy, J., Kapustina, A., Muhina, N., & Irving, S. (1998). Association of alcohol consumption to mortality in middle-aged U.S. and Russian men and women. *Annals of Epidemiology, 8,* 147–153.

Douglas, M. (1992). *Risk and blame: Essays in cultural theory.* London: Routledge.

Douglas, M., & Wildavsky, A. B. (1982). *Risk and culture. An essay on the selection of technical and environmental dangers.* Berkeley: University of California Press.

Faggiano, F., Partanen, T., Kogevinas, M., & Boffeta, P. (1997). Socioeconomic differences in cancer incidence and mortality. In M. Kogevinas, N. Pearce, M. Susser, & P. Boffeta (Eds.), *Social inequalities in cancer* (pp. 65–176). Lyon: International Agency for Research on Cancer.

Fekjaer, H. O. (1993). *Alcohol and illicit drugs: Myths and realities.* Colombo, Sri Lanka: International Order of Good Templars, Alcohol and Drug Information Centre.

Flaminio, D. (1989). *Drinking and driving: Cultural aspects and practical implications.* Dissertation. Triest, Italy: University of Trieste Press.

Fleming, C. M., & Manson, S. M. (1990). Native American women. In R. C. Engs (Ed.), *Women: Alcohol and other drugs* (pp. 143–148). Dubuque, IA: Kendall/Hunt Publishing Company.

Flynn, J., Slovic, P., & Mertz, C. K. (1994). Gender, race, and perception of environmental health risks. *Risk Analysis, 14,* 1101–1108.

Fromme, K., Katz, E. C., & Rivet, K. (1997). Outcome expectancies and risk-taking behavior. *Cognitive Therapy and Research, 21,* 421–442.

Gracey, M. (1998). Substance misuse in Aboriginal Australians. *Addiction Biology, 3,* 9–46.

Gray, D., & Chickritz, T. (2000). Regional variation in alcohol consumption in the Northern Territory. *Australian and New Zealand Journal of Public Health, 24,* 35–38.

Hartman, J. (1990). The Delft bicycle network. In R. Tolley (Ed.), *The greening of urban transport: Planning for walking and cycling in Western cities.* London: Bellhaven Press.

Heath, D. B. (1995). *International handbook on alcohol and culture.* Westport, CT: Greenwood.

Heath, D. B. (2000). *Drinking occasions. Comparative perspectives on alcohol and culture.* Philadelphia, PA: Brunner/Mazel.

Heath, D. B. (2001). Culture and substance abuse. *Cultural Psychiatry: International Perspectives, 24,* 479–495.

Hennen, J. R., & Knudten, R. D. (2001). A lifestyle analysis of the elderly: Perceptions of risk, fear, and vulnerability. *Illness, Crisis & Loss, 9,* 190–208.

Huyink, W. (1987). Cycling policy in the city of Groningen. Traffic Department of Groningen.

International Center for Alcohol Policies (ICAP) (1998). *Drinking age limits* (Report No. 4). Washington, DC: Author.

ICAP (1999). *Government policies on alcohol and pregnancy* (Report No. 6). Washington, DC: Author.

ICAP (2000). *Who are the abstainers?* (Report No. 8). Washington, DC: Author.

ICAP (2001). *Alcohol and "special populations": Biological vulnerability* (Report No. 10). Washington, DC: Author.

Jones, J. H. (1993). *Bad blood. The Tuskegee syphilis experiment* (2nd ed.). New York: The Free Press.

Koopmans, J. R., Slutske, W. S., van Baal, G. C. M., & Boomsma, D. I. (1999). The influence of religion on alcohol use initiation: Evidence for genotype X environment interaction. *Behavior Genetics, 29,* 445–453.

Kreitman, N. (1986). Alcohol consumption and the preventive paradox. *British Journal of Addiction, 81,* 353–363.

La Fée Verte Absinthe House. (2003). *Les Beaux Arts.* Retrieved August 21, 2003, from http://www.feeverte.net.

Ma, G. X., Toubbeh, J., Cline, J., & Chisholm, A. (2002). Model for fetal alcohol syndrome prevention in Native American population. In G. X. Ma & G. Henderson (Eds.), *Ethnicity and substance abuse: Prevention and intervention* (pp. 284–295). Springfield, IL: Charles C. Thomas Publisher Ltd.

MacAndrew, C., & Edgerton, R. E. (1969). *Drunken comportment.* Chicago: Aldine.

Macdonald, D., & Molamu, L. (1999). From pleasure to pain: A social history of Basarwa/San alcohol use in Botswana. In S. Peele & M. Grant (Eds.), *Alcohol and pleasure: A health perspective* (pp. 73–86). Philadelphia, PA: Brunner/Mazel.

Madsen, W., & Madsen, C. (1979). The cultural structure of Mexican drinking behavior. In M. Marshall (Ed.), *Beliefs, behaviors, and alcoholic beverages* (pp. 38–54). Ann Arbor: The University of Michigan Press.

Mäkëla, K. (1983). The uses of alcohol and their cultural regulation. *Acta Sociologica, 26,* 21–31.

Marmot, M., Shipley, M. J., & Rose, G. (1984). Inequalities in death—specific explanations of a general pattern? *Lancet, I,* 1003–1006.

Marshall, M. (Ed.). (1979). *Beliefs, behaviors, and alcoholic beverages: A cross-cultural survey.* Ann Arbor: The University of Michigan Press.

Marteau, T., & Richards, M. (Eds.). (1999). *The troubled helix.* Cambridge, UK: Cambridge University Press.

May, P. A., Brooke, L., Gossage, J. P., Croxford, J., Adams, C., Jones, K. L., et al. (2000). Epidemiology of fetal alcohol syndrome in a South African community in the Western Cape Province. *American Journal of Public Health, 90,* 1905–1912.

Midanik, L. T., & Clark, W. B. (1994). The demographic distribution of U.S. drinking patterns in 1990: Description and trends from 1984. *American Journal of Public Health, 84,* 1218–1222.

Monaghan, L., Bloor, M., Dobash, R. P., & Dobash, R. E. (2000). Drug-taking, "risk boundaries" and social identity: Bodybuilders talk about ephedrine and nubain. *Sociological Research Online, 5* .

Murray, C. J. L., & Lopez, A. D. (1996). Quantifying the burden of disease and injury attributable to ten major risk factors. In C. J. L. Murray & A. D. Lopez (Eds.), *The global burden of disease: A comprehensive assessment of mortality and disability from diseases, injuries, and risk factors in 1990 and projected to 2020.* Boston: Harvard School of Public Health.

Musto, D. F. (1996). Alcohol in American history. *Scientific American, 274,* 78–83.

National Center for Health Services. (1998). *Health, United States, with socioeconomic status and health chartbook.* Hyattsville, MD: Public Health Service.

National Health & Medical Research Council. (2001). *Australian alcohol guidelines: Health risks and benefits.* Canberra: Author.

Nelson, D. E., Moon, R. W., Holtzman, D., Smith, P., & Siegel, P. Z. (1997). Patterns of health risk behaviors for chronic disease: A comparison between adolescent and adult American Indians living on or near reservations in Montana. *Journal of Adolescent Health, 21,* 25–32.

O'Leary, C. (2002). *Fetal alcohol syndrome: A literature review.* Canberra, Australia: Commonwealth Department on Health and Aging.

Palosuo, H. (2000). Health-related lifestyles and alienation in Moscow and Helsinki. *Social Science & Medicine, 51,* 1325–1341.

Patel, V. (2001). Poverty, inequality and mental health in developing countries. In D. Leon & G. Walt (Eds.), *Poverty, inequality and health: An international perspective* (pp. 247–282). Oxford, UK: Oxford University Press.

Petrie, K. J., Siverstsen, B., Hysing, M., Broadbent, E., Moss-Morris, R., Eriksen, H. R., et al. (2001). Thoroughly modern worries. The relationship of worries about modernity to reported symptoms, health and medical care utilization. *Journal of Psychosomatic Research, 51,* 395–401.

Pittman, D. J. (1967). International overview: Social and cultural factors in drinking patterns, pathological and nonpathological. In D. J. Pittman (Ed.), *Alcoholism* (pp. 3–22). New York: Harper & Row.

Plant, M., & Plant, M. (1992). *Risk-takers: Alcohol, drugs, sex and youth.* London: Tavistock/Routledge.

Plant, M. L., Abel, E. L., & Guerri, C. (1999). Alcohol and pregnancy. In I. Macdonald (Ed.), *Health issues related to alcohol consumption* (pp. 181–213). Oxford, UK: Blackwell Science Ltd.

Poldrugo, F., & Flaminio, D. (1990). Alcohol and driving: An underestimated problem in Italy. *Alcoholism: Clinical and Experimental Research, 14,* 329.

Preston, B. (1990). The safety of walking and cycling in different countries. In R. Tolley (Ed.), *The greening of urban transport: Planning for walking and cycling in Western countries* (pp. 49–52). London: Bellhaven Press.

Racz, J., Vingender, I., Schaffer, L., & Pakozdi, L. (Eds.). (1999). *Role of major addictions (alcoholism, smoking, drug abuse) in morbidity, mortality and decrease of population in Hungary: Statistical analysis for the Parliament 1998.* Budapest, Hungary: National Institute of Alcohology.

Regidor, E., Gutierrez-Fisac, J. L., Calle, M. E., Navarro, P., & Dominguez, V. (2001). Trends in cigarette smoking in Spain by social class. *Preventive Medicine: An International Journal Devoted to Practice and Theory, 33,* 241–248.

Room, R., & Mäkelä, K. (2000). Typologies of the cultural position of drinking. *Journal of Studies on Alcohol, 61,* 475–483.

Rorabaugh, W. (1979). *Alcoholic republic: An American tradition.* New York: Oxford University Press.

Royal, D. (2000a). *Report and ethnic group comparisons national surveys of drinking and driving—attitudes and behavior—1993, 1995, and 1997: Findings* (Vol. 1). Washington, DC: U.S. Department of Transportation, National Highway Traffic Safety Administration.

Royal, D. (2000b). *Report and ethnic group comparisons national surveys of drinking and driving—attitudes and behavior—1993, 1995, and 1997: Methods Report (Vol. 2).* Washington, DC: U.S. Department of Transportation, National Highway Traffic Safety Administration.

Royal College of Obstetricians and Gynaecologists (RCOG). (1999). Alcohol consumption in pregnancy (RCOG Guideline No. 9). London: Author.

Rozin, P., & Singh, L. (1999). The moralization of cigarette smoking in the United States. *Journal of Consumer Psychology, 8,* 339–342.

Sachdev, P. S. (1990). Behavioral factors affecting physical health of the New Zealand Maori. *Science and Social Medicine, 30,* 431–440.

Schmidt, L., & Room, R. (1999). Cross-cultural applicability in international classifications and research on alcohol dependence. *Journal of Studies on Alcohol, 60,* 448–462.

Sjöberg, L. (1998). World views, political attitudes and risk perception. *Risk: Health, Safety and Environment, 9,* 137–152.

Slovic, P. (1999). Trust, emotion, sex, politics, and science: Surveying the risk-assessment battlefield. *Risk Analysis, 19,* 689–701.

Snortum, J. (1990). Drinking-driving compliance in Great Britain: The role of law as a "threat" and as a "moral eye-opener." *Journal of Criminal Justice, 18,* 475–489.

Stronks, K., van de Mheen, H. D., Looman, C. W. N., & Mackenbach, J. P. (1997). Cultural, material, and psychosocial correlates of the socioeconomic gradient in smoking behavior among adults. *Preventive Medicine: An International Journal Devoted to Practice and Theory, 26,* 754–766.

Sturm, R. (2002). The effects of obesity, smoking, and drinking on medical problems and costs. *Health Affairs, 21,* 245–253.

Substance Abuse & Mental Health Service Administration (2002). American Indians/ Alaska Natives and substance abuse. *Prevention Alert, 5.*

ten Grotenhuis, D. (1986). *The Delft Cycle Plan.* Groningen: Netherlands Center for Research and Contract Standardization in Civil and Traffic Engineering.

Trotter, R. T. I. (1985). Folk medicine in the Southwest: Myths and medical facts. *Postgraduate Medicine, 78,* 167–179.

Trotter, R. T. I. (1991). A survey of four illnesses and their relationship to intracultural variation in a Mexican-American community. *American Anthropologist, 93,* 115–125.

U.S. Bureau of Census. (2003). *International Data Base.* Retrieved August 21, 2003, from http://www.census.gov/ipc/www/idbnew.html.

Viljoen, D. (1999). Fetal alcohol syndrome. *South African Medical Journal, 89,* 958–960.

Wadsworth, M. (1999). Early life. In M. Marmot & R. Wilkinson (Eds.), *Social determinants of health* (pp. 44–63). New York: Oxford University Press.

Wechsler, H., Lee, J., Nelson, T., & Lee, H. (2001). Drinking levels, alcohol problems and secondhand effects in substance-free college residences: Results of a national survey. *Journal of Studies on Alcohol, 66,* 23–31.

World Advertising Research Center (WARC). (2003). *World Drink Trends: 2003.* Henley-on-Thames, Oxfordshire, UK: Author.

The World Bank/International Bank for Reconstruction and Development. (2000). *World development indicators 2000.* Washington, DC: Author.

The World Bank/International Bank for Reconstruction and Development. (2001). *World development report 2000/2001: Attacking poverty.* New York: Oxford University Press.

World Health Organization (WHO). (2000). *New healthy life expectancy rankings.* Geneva: Author.

Zielinski, A. (1994). Polish culture: Dry or wet? *Contemporary Drug Problems, 21,* 329–340.

Chapter 3

It's Not Only the Numbers That Count: Assessing Risk and Benefit

"Drink or three a day deters dementia, study concludes"

Seattle Times *(Ross, 2002)*

"Just one drink a week can lower stroke risk in men, biggest study yet reports"

Seattle Times *(Greenberg, 1999)*

"Conflicting breast cancer studies creating unsettling uncertainties"

New York Times *(Lewin, 2001)*

Health news is big news. Coverage of scientific and health advances is increasing, and many such findings are reported as front-page news (Nelkin, 1995). The health information that we receive from media reports plays an important role in shaping our perceptions and our knowledge about health. In a U.S. survey about the impact of health news, 75% of survey respondents reported paying a "moderate amount" or a "great deal" of attention to medical and health news reported by the media, and nearly half said they had changed their behavior as a result of a media report of medical or health news (Johnson, 1998). Clearly, the public is interested in knowing more about the results of medical research and is eager to apply it to their own lives. Nevertheless, when it comes to understanding these reports, we are often at a loss. What do the statements in these reports mean, and where do they come from?

Consider, for example, a press release from the American Cancer Society, which states that "recent studies leave little doubt that alcohol intake increases breast cancer risk . . . just one to two drinks can increase risk for some women" (American Cancer Society, 2001). The reader is left asking, "If alcohol increases risk, *how much* does it increase the risk? Which women are affected the most?" Even when a media report includes numbers, readers may still wonder exactly what the numbers signify. For example, a recent Associated Press report on the association of drinking to the development of dementia noted that "people who drank between one and three drinks a day . . . had a 42 percent lower risk of developing dementia than the non-drinkers. Those who weren't daily drinkers but had more than one drink per week had a 25 percent lower risk and those who drank less than a glass a week were 18 percent less likely than nondrinkers to develop dementia" (Ross, 2002). But what does it mean to be at 25% lower risk, and how did scientists come up with these numbers?

Although the concepts of risk and probability of harm are the same for different kinds of risks, the ways in which risks and benefits are measured can vary widely across scientific disciplines. Different types of risks are assessed in different ways. Technological risks are assessed using principles from safety and engineering disciplines. This area of risk assessment and risk management is an active one, encompassing such issues as nuclear power plants and genetically engineered foods. Risks from pharmaceuticals and environmental contaminants are assessed with principles of toxicology, which often involve controlled experiments with animals. Financial risks, such as the risks arising from the stock market, involve economic forecasting.

To effectively use the information about health risks that we learn from television, the newspaper, or our own physicians, we should understand the principles that underlie research into these risks. This chapter provides a brief review of the methods that are used to study health outcomes, including the outcomes of alcohol consumption, and addresses such questions as:

- What do the risk "numbers" that we read about in the newspaper signify?
- How are these numbers derived from research studies, and how are these studies conducted?
- Given inconsistent findings on risks, how can we interpret the numbers and figure out how to use them?

THE ROLE OF BASIC RESEARCH

"Basic" research usually refers to research that investigates chemical or biological processes. Such research is normally done either with whole, living animals (in vivo) or with biological samples (in vitro). Basic research is used to study phenomena that cannot be examined practically or ethically in humans, or to identify the biological mechanisms that underlie the development of human diseases. For example, basic laboratory research on alcohol has examined:

- The effects of chronic alcohol abuse on the body's ability to process nutrients, potentially negating the beneficial effects of "healthy" diets on decreasing risk for certain cancers (National Institute on Alcohol Abuse and Alcoholism, 1993);
- The association of alcohol abuse and immune suppression, making abusers more susceptible to infectious diseases;
- The effects of alcohol on platelet function and arterial narrowing, which play a role in protecting the heart (National Institute on Alcohol Abuse and Alcoholism, 1999);
- The effects of maternal alcohol use on birth defects (Maier & West, 2001).

An important characteristic of animal studies is the experimenter's control over all conditions of the study, enabling researchers to study alcohol effects at precise doses without needing to worry about extraneous factors that might affect the results. Of course, extrapolating the results of animal studies to humans involves dealing with species differences in alcohol metabolism and a host of other factors. Nevertheless, basic research has provided crucial insights into the effects of alcohol and the mechanisms whereby alcohol exerts these effects.

EPIDEMIOLOGIC RESEARCH

Health risks, such as those posed by drinking, are generally studied using principles and methods of epidemiology, which is the study of the distribution and determinants of diseases in populations. An important part of this definition is that it applies to populations or groups of people instead of to individuals. Results of epidemiologic research are used to draw conclusions about target populations, not individuals (Coggon, Rose, & Barker, 1997). Whereas some other scientific disciplines depend on controlled experiments to study the etiology, or origins, of certain phenomena, epidemiology is largely observational; that is, in epidemiologic research, we observe the world as it is instead of construct a controlled environment. This is both the strength and weakness of epidemiology. Studying people as they actually live in the real world means that what we observe is what happens naturally over the course of living. At the same time, real life is messy, making it extremely difficult for epidemiologists to disentangle the interrelated threads that contribute to health conditions.

Describing the Health of a Population: Descriptive Epidemiology

Descriptive epidemiology is concerned with describing the general characteristics of a disease or health condition, with particular reference to person, place, and time (Hennekens & Buring, 1987; Schoenbach & Rosamond, 2000). Examples of descriptive epidemiology include:

- Routine analyses of vital statistics such as births and deaths;
- Surveillance of conditions to report to health authorities, such as certain infectious diseases;

- Periodic surveys of health status and health care utilization;
- Census data.

Information from descriptive studies is essential to determine which segments of the population are most affected by health conditions and to help target resources, education, and prevention programs to the appropriate subgroups (Hennekens & Buring, 1987). This descriptive information supplies important baseline data and provides a context for developing hypotheses, designing studies, and interpreting results (Schoenbach & Rosamond, 2000).

Numbers alone are rarely meaningful. For example, knowing that 50,000 cases of chicken pox occur among children in Freedonia each year doesn't tell us much unless we know the actual population of Freedonia. Do 50,000 cases represent a small proportion of the population or a large proportion? For this reason, epidemiologic research focuses on *rates* instead of numbers. A rate reflects the number of cases of the disease (the numerator) divided by the number of individuals in the relevant population (the denominator), over a specified period during which the outcomes occur. The two basic rates used in epidemiologic studies are:

> *Incidence:* the rate at which new cases of the disease (or condition) occur in a population during a specified period;
> *Prevalence:* the proportion of a population that has the disease (or condition) at a particular time point; an appropriate measure for relatively stable conditions.

For example, suppose that 1 million children under the age of 12 lived in Freedonia in 2001, and 1,000 children contracted chicken pox during that year. The *incidence* of chicken pox is then $1,000/1,000,000 = 1$ case per 1,000 children per year. If 85,000 Freedonian children have asthma at a specific time point (e.g., at the time of a health survey), the *prevalence* of asthma is 85/1,000. (Because many health conditions are relatively rare, and because of the difficulty in managing decimal points, epidemiologists often present rates in terms of the number per 100,000 people/year. The rate of chicken pox in Freedonian children would be described as 100 cases per 100,000 children/year.)

When only raw numbers are presented, without reference to an underlying population (so-called "floating numerators" [Coggon, Rose, & Barker, 1997]), they may be interesting but are often misleading. For example, annual statistics on treatment for decompression sickness (DCS) among scuba divers showed that in 2001, 192 of these diving injuries occurred in the Caribbean and 18 in the Pacific Islands (Divers Alert Network, 2003). Does this mean that it is more dangerous to dive in the Caribbean than in the Pacific? This is not the case when we consider that many more divers travel to the Caribbean for diving vacations than to the islands in the Pacific. Thus, many more injuries would be expected because of the sheer numbers involved.

Investigating the Determinants of Health Outcomes: Analytic Epidemiology

Going beyond basic descriptions of health characteristics of a population, analytic epidemiology focuses on identifying *associations* between *exposures* and *outcomes* (Gerstman, 1998; Hennekens & Buring, 1987; Schoenbach & Rosamond, 2000). Theories of disease etiology or clues from descriptive studies give rise to hypotheses about the relationship of exposure to disease that can be tested. The dividing line between descriptive and analytic methods is blurred, given that many studies include both descriptive and analytic aspects, but in general, hypothesis testing is the hallmark of the analytic study.

Exposure: Any explanatory variable that might be related to the disease or condition under study. Although the term implies biological agents, it can represent any explanatory variable, including biological, behavioral, or environmental factors (Gerstman, 1998).

Disease: A physical or psychological dysfunction, or any health-related outcome under study. Again, although this term implies a defined medical condition, it is used in epidemiology to refer to any outcome under study (Gerstman, 1998).

Association: A relationship or statistical dependence between the exposure and disease. Exposure and disease are associated if changing the value of one changes the distribution of the other. A *positive association* exists when higher levels of exposure are associated with increased levels of a disease; a *negative association* exists when higher levels of exposure predict a decrease in the outcome (Gerstman, 1998; Last, 2001).

Risk factor: An exposure that is associated with increased risk of disease (Last, 2001).

The increasingly voluminous research on the relationship between moderate drinking and coronary heart disease offers a useful example. Descriptive studies tell us about the disease (i.e., rates of heart disease in various countries, by gender and age) and about the exposure (i.e., rates of drinking and abstention, by gender and age). We might notice, as have many others, that rates of heart disease, and rates of drinking, differ across countries. The next step is to design an analytic study to examine the *association* of drinking to heart disease. Our basic approach involves:

1. Measuring the occurrence of heart disease among drinkers and non-drinkers (In reality, we would use several groups of drinkers—light, moderate, and heavy—but this example is simplified.)
2. Comparing the occurrence of heart disease in the two groups
3. Quantifying this comparison with a measure of association (Schoenbach & Rosamund, 2000)

Measures of Risk, Odds, and Association

In epidemiology, risk refers to the probability that an outcome will occur within a certain time interval (Schoenbach & Rosamond, 2000). For example, we may hear that an American woman's risk of developing breast cancer in her lifetime (if she lives to age 85 without dying of something else) is 1 in 8 (Ries et al., 2003), or that the risk of being injured in an automobile accident is 109 per 100 million miles driven (National Highway Traffic Safety Administration, 2001).

In order to examine associations between exposures and outcomes, we look at the *relative risk,* which is the risk for people exposed to the factor in question compared with the risk among those not exposed:

$$\text{Relative risk} = \frac{\text{(risk among the exposed)}}{\text{(risk among the unexposed)}}$$

The relative risk expresses how much more or less likely the outcome is to occur in people with the exposure. A relative risk of 1 indicates that the risk is the same in both groups; so there is no association of exposure and outcome. A relative risk greater than 1 indicates that exposed people are more likely to develop the outcome (a positive association), while a relative risk of less than 1 indicates that exposed people are less likely to develop the outcome (a negative association). For example, a relative risk of 2 indicates that exposed people are twice as likely to develop the outcome; a relative risk of 1.2 indicates that exposed people are 20% *more* likely to develop the outcome; and a relative risk of .6 indicates that exposed people are 40% *less* likely to develop the outcome.

In a study of respiratory problems (Eagan, Gulsvik, Eide, & Bakke, 2002), a random sample of residents of western Norway were mailed a questionnaire that asked about occupational exposure to airborne dust, fumes, asbestos, and quartz, as well as about smoking and respiratory symptoms. A second questionnaire was sent 11 years later with similar questions. Among people who had no exposure at the baseline measurement, the rate of chronic bronchitis symptoms (i.e., chronic cough plus phlegm cough) was 4.1%; among people exposed to asbestos, the rate was 10.6%. The relative risk for asbestos exposure is (10.6/100) divided by (4.1/100) = 2.56, indicating that people exposed to asbestos were two and a half times more likely to develop these symptoms than those who were not exposed to asbestos.

To investigate back injuries among firefighters, researchers classified 1652 firefighters without prior back injury into three groups based on five measures of strength and fitness. Over the next 4 years, back injuries occurred in 7.1% of the low-fitness group, 3.2% of the moderate fitness group, and .8% of the high-fitness group. The relative risk for moderate fitness, compared with low fitness, is (3.2/100) divided by (7.1/100) = .45, indicating that moderately fit firefighters were 55% less likely to suffer a back injury than less fit firefighters (Cady, Bischoff, O'Connell, Thomas, & Allan, 1979).

Note that a large *relative* risk can be found in conjunction with a small *absolute* risk, and vice versa. For example, heavy alcohol consumption approximately triples the risk of developing esophageal cancer. However, the absolute risk of esophageal cancer remains small—4 per 100,000 per year in the U.S. general population. Even tripled, this risk is still small. Conversely, a small relative risk can have large effects when combined with a large absolute risk. Recent reports suggest that the relative risk for drinking and breast cancer is 1.2–1.3, a much smaller relative risk than that of drinking and esophageal cancer; however, the absolute risk of breast cancer is much larger than that of esophageal cancer (114/100,000). Therefore, a smaller increase in risk due to drinking (20–30%) actually gives rise to more actual cases of cancer. That is, "a large number of people at a small risk may give rise to more cases of disease than the small number who are at a high risk" (Rose, 1985).

In some studies, as described next, the rates of disease in people with and without a risk factor cannot be calculated. In these studies, an alternative measure of association is used: the *odds ratio*. Odds are familiar to those who bet on horses or gamble with dice. The odds of an event occurring are equal to the ratio of the probability that it will occur to the probability that it will not. Thus,

$$\text{Odds} = \frac{\text{p(event occurs)}}{\text{p(event does not occur)}}$$

and equivalently,

$$\frac{\text{p(event occurs)}}{1 - \text{p(event occur)}}$$

For example, the probability of rolling a die and getting a six is 1/6 = .167. The odds of rolling a six are 1/5. Note that the odds are always larger than the risk, but for very low probability events, the odds and the risk are nearly equal. For example, if the risk of a particular outcome is only 1 in 10,000, the risk will be .0001 while the odds will be .00010001.

The *odds ratio* is simply the ratio of two odds. In epidemiologic research, this can be the odds of a particular outcome (such as developing the disease) among the exposed compared with the odds of that outcome among the unexposed. For diseases with low prevalence, the odds ratio approximates the relative risk. Both the odds ratio and the relative risk are measures of association; that is, they quantify the strength of the relationship between the exposure and the outcome.

Types of Studies in Epidemiology

Case Series

A *case report* is a clinical description of an unusual medical occurrence, and a *case series* is a set of individual case reports documenting the same occurrence

(Hennekens & Buring, 1987). In case series, exposure histories are described in people with the same injury or illness. Case reports and case series are descriptive studies that can lead to identification of new diseases or to the discovery of an epidemic of existing disease.

Case Series Example

In 1980 and 1981, several cases of previously healthy young men with rare forms of pneumonia and cancer were reported in Los Angeles. The appearance of these diseases was unusual, given that these diseases were seen almost exclusively in older people and those with suppressed immune systems (Gottlieb et al., 1981). These reports led to a surveillance program initiated by the U.S. Centers for Disease Control, which quickly found that most of these new cases were homosexual men. Subsequent reports of similar conditions in intravenous drug abusers and recipients of blood transfusions pointed to blood-borne transmission of the new disease. These findings provided crucial clues that were used to design studies to identify the risk factors for the disease that came to be called AIDS (Hennekens & Buring, 1987).

Although case series can provide clues about risk factors, they cannot demonstrate an association between exposure and outcome because calculating an association requires that both the exposure and the disease vary. A common error in research on drinking and events such as injuries and crime is to interpret the results of case series as demonstrating an *association* of drinking to the event. For example, writings on drinking and crime nearly always include percentages of different kinds of criminal events in which alcohol is found. The authors of these treatises point to these percentages as demonstrations that drinking is "associated" with crime—an incorrect interpretation. Knowing the proportion of offenders who were drinking at the time of the crime is not meaningful unless we know the proportion of drinkers among people who did *not* commit crimes; if these proportions are the same, then there is no association of drinking to crime.

Sometimes, case series can contribute valuable information about the etiology of an event or condition (Cummings & Weiss, 1998). A case series does have an implied control group (i.e., everyone else in the population from which the cases were derived). The level of exposure in the cases can be so out of the range of what is known about the population that it is somewhat clear that the exposure is related to the outcome. The classic example is Sir Percivall Pott's 18th-century description of scrotal cancer, which he called "the chimney-sweeper's cancer" because nearly all the cases he saw were in chimney sweeps (Pott, 1778). Because it was clear that the majority of the general population were not chimney sweeps, there was an implied association between chimney sweeping and scrotal cancer. Later research identified soot as the culprit.

Some commentators have used similar logic in the case of drinking and crime, reasoning that drinking appears in such a large proportion of crimes that it is unlikely that a similar proportion of the general population would be drinking at a particular time. Evans notes, however, that in the west of Scotland, the proportion of offenders who were intoxicated at the time of their offense corresponds with the proportion of men expected to be intoxicated at similar times (Evans, 1986). Moreover, drinking among convicted offenders at the time of the offense is no greater than would be expected given their typical drinking patterns (Kalish, 1983; Ladouceur & Temple, 1985). Data from the U.S. Bureau of Justice Statistics show that one-third of state prison inmates reported drinking heavily just before they committed the offense for which they were incarcerated, but 20% of all inmates reported that they drank very heavily every day of the entire year before entering prison (Greenfield, 1998). Thus, the occurrence of drinking in criminal events does not appear to be substantially different from the occurrence of drinking in the underlying population at risk for committing crimes.

Cross-Sectional Studies

A *cross-sectional study,* also called a prevalence study or a survey study, represents a snapshot of a population at a particular time point. In this kind of study, people are surveyed about their health status, including various exposures and diseases. Cross-sectional studies include, for example, periodic national surveys of health status by federal agencies, as well as targeted surveys of particular health conditions. The results of these studies provide information about the occurrence of risk factors and health outcomes in relation to sociodemographic variables such as age, gender, and race.

Note that a cross-sectional study assesses only current diseases and exposures, and thus cannot usually distinguish whether the exposure or the disease came first. For this reason, cross-sectional studies usually cannot be used to determine risk factors for disease. For example, a cross-sectional survey in Japan reported that people who exercised regularly were about half as likely to have difficulty falling asleep as nonexercisers (Kim et al., 1999). Does this mean that physical activity promotes better sleep? Perhaps, but with this study, we don't know whether the lack of physical activity preceded or followed the beginning of sleep problems. People who have difficulty sleeping may decrease their physical exercise due to lack of energy.

Cross-sectional studies of alcohol and criminal activity usually show that heavier drinkers are more likely to have engaged in criminal behavior, and that prison populations have higher rates of heavy drinking, drinking problems, and alcohol disorders than the general population (Collins, 1993; Graham, Schmidt, & Gillis, 1996). Nevertheless, disentangling the directionality of this association is difficult. Drinking may lead to criminal activity, or criminality may precede alcohol problems (Goodwin, Crane, & Guze, 1971; Pittman & Gordon, 1958; White, 1997).

Strengths and Weaknesses of Cross-Sectional Studies

Strengths

- Useful for describing the characteristics of a population;
- Good for assessing the prevalence of chronic problems;
- If the samples are chosen carefully, the results can be generalized to the population.

Weaknesses

- Cannot establish the temporal relationship of exposures and outcomes;
- May not capture prevalence of uncommon exposures or rare outcomes;
- Susceptible to selection bias and recall bias (defined later in this chapter).

Ecological Studies

An *ecological study,* also known as an aggregate study or correlational study, uses data from groups of people or entities rather than from individuals. In an ecological study, exposures and outcomes are measured at the level of a community, political entity, or group, and often uses routinely collected vital statistics (Schoenbach & Rosamond, 2000). A study that compares rates across countries or regions is an ecological study, as are studies that compare rates over time in a single population. Ecological studies have shown, for example, that rates of colon cancer are higher in countries with high meat consumption (Armstrong & Doll, 1975), and that rates of esophageal cancer are higher in areas with poor-quality well water (Yokokawa et al., 1999).

Ecological Study Example

The U.S. is one of 84 countries worldwide that allows capital punishment for certain crimes. Currently, 38 states have the death penalty. A recent analysis reported in the *New York Times* found that homicide rates in states with the death penalty were higher than rates in states without the death penalty. Over the last 20 years, the homicide rate in death penalty states has been 48 to 100% higher than in states with no death penalty, suggesting that the threat of the death penalty does not deter crime (Bonner & Fessenden, 2000).

Unquestionably, the best known ecological association in the alcohol literature is the relationship between alcohol consumption and heart disease, as reflected in the "French paradox": Despite high fat consumption, the French enjoy low rates of heart disease. This phenomenon has been explained by reference to a protective effect of alcohol (in this case, particularly red wine) on the cardiovascular system. Ecological studies tend to show that countries with a high consumption of red wine have lower rates of heart disease (Rimm, Klatsky, Grobbee, & Stampfer, 1996).

An ecological study is sometimes considered a descriptive study (Hennekens & Buring, 1987), and is sometimes classified as "incomplete" because of information missing on some relevant factors (Kleinbaum, Kupper, & Morgenstern, 1982). In this type of study, the missing information is at the level of the individual, making it impossible to link exposure and disease in the same person. Taking the example of meat consumption and colon cancer, it is not possible to tell whether the people who consume more meat are the ones who develop the disease. Inferring exposure–disease relationships *within* individuals from group-level measures is called the *ecological fallacy*. Note that this fallacy does not arise from the ecological method itself but only from drawing individual-level conclusions from population-level data (Schoenbach & Rosamond, 2000).

Ecological studies are also particularly prone to the effects of unmeasured and uncontrolled variables that can explain the relationship between the exposure and disease. (These *confounding variables* are discussed later in this chapter.) Countries, regions, and groups of people vary in many ways other than the exposure being studied, and these variations can account for variations in disease frequency. For example, people in Mediterranean countries, who have high alcohol consumption and low rates of heart disease, also have different eating patterns, including drinking alcohol with meals, low consumption of saturated fats, and high consumption of fruits and vegetables. These dietary factors, rather than alcohol consumption, may be responsible for lower rates of cardiovascular disease in this population.

Studies of alcohol and crime illustrate the distinction between the ecological fallacy and the role of confounding variables. Population-level analyses show that in the U.S., regions with higher per capita alcohol consumption also have higher rates of violent crime (Parker & Cartmill, 1998; Parker & Rebhun, 1995). Inferring that alcohol makes people become violent is an example of the ecological fallacy because we cannot tell whether the people who are drinking are the same people who are committing the crimes. We know that for some interpersonal crimes, alcohol is most strongly involved in victimization. People who are drinking may be less able to protect themselves and to exercise sound judgment, and might be sufficiently obnoxious to provoke violence (Collins & Messerschmidt, 1993). Thus, it is quite possible that increases in crime follow increases in alcohol consumption because of more drinking among victims instead of among perpetrators.

Moreover, other variables besides drinking may be responsible for violent crime. For example, drinking is closely related to social interaction. When drinking levels decrease, the frequency of social interaction is also reduced, with a resulting decrease in the probability of interpersonal crime. Alcohol may be associated with violence by attracting offenders and victims to high-risk environments, or by increasing the number of male gatherings (Lipsey, Wilson, Cohen, & Derzon, 1997). For example, criminologists have written about a "routine activity" approach to crime, in which criminal acts require space and time convergence of likely offenders and suitable targets, as well as the absence of capable guardians against crime (Cohen & Felson, 1979). Drinking activities can contribute to this convergence by attracting people to certain locations, increasing the frequency of interactions with others, and making people more vulnerable to attack (Parker & Cartmill, 1998; Parker & Rebhun, 1995). Therefore, it may not be drinking per se that reduces or increases levels of crime, but other common cause factors that are associated with both drinking and crime.

Strengths and Weaknesses of Ecological Studies

Strengths

- Often can be done quickly and inexpensively with existing data;
- Can assess effects of group-level factors, for example, laws or services (Schoenbach & Rosamond, 2000).

Weaknesses

- Cannot infer individual characteristics from group-level measures (ecological fallacy);
- Unmeasured differences between groups can be responsible for different levels of the outcome.

Case–Control Studies

The *case–control* design has been called the most significant innovation in epidemiology of the 20th century. In this design, two groups of people are studied: people who have the condition or outcome of interest (cases) and people who are free of the condition (controls). Exposures are then measured and compared between cases and controls to identify exposures that might explain why some people have the condition and some do not. For example, in Doll and Hill's (1950) influential study of smoking and lung cancer, the cases were 1,465 patients who were admitted to London hospitals with a new diagnosis of lung cancer, and the controls were patients who were hospitalized with other disorders. Cases and controls were interviewed concerning smoking habits, and the results showed that patients with lung cancer were nine times more likely to be smokers than were patients without cancer.

Case–Control Study Example

Bicycling is a leading cause of recreational injuries in the U.S., and elevated blood alcohol concentrations (BACs) are found in 32% of people who die of bicycling injuries. To assess the association of drinking with bicycling injury, researchers obtained results of blood alcohol tests of bicyclists who were injured seriously or fatally. The researchers then visited the sites at which the bicyclists were injured, and then administered roadside surveys and blood alcohol tests to passing bicyclists. A positive BAC was detected in 24% of the fatally injured bicyclists, 9% of the seriously injured bicyclists, and 3% of the uninjured bicyclists. The odds of being injured were 10 times greater for bicyclists with BACs above 0.08 than for bicyclists with BACs below 0.02 (Li, Baker, Smialek, & Soderstrom, 2001).

Because case–control studies can be conducted somewhat quickly and cheaply, they are often used in initial investigations of suspected associations of exposures and diseases. A major advantage of the case–control method is its efficiency for studying rare conditions. For example, a researcher studying ALS (amyotrophic lateral sclerosis, or Lou Gehrig's disease) in the general population would have to sift through 100,000 people in order to find two people with the disease. With a case–control study, the researcher could instead enroll all new cases of ALS from hospitals and physicians' offices to collect a sufficient number of cases for study. Moreover, the researcher can investigate the effect of several different exposures in the same study, as long as the exposures are relatively common; rare exposures will not be present in sufficient numbers to study effectively.

The validity of a case–control study depends on careful selection of cases and controls. Cases enrolled in the study must be typical of cases in the population, and controls must be typical of people in the population who do not have the outcome of interest (Gerstman, 1998). If cases or controls are not representative of the underlying populations, the association of exposure to outcome will be inaccurate. For example, in Doll and Hill's study of smoking and lung cancer, controls were patients hospitalized for diseases other than lung cancer. Because smoking is associated with a number of different diseases, hospitalized people generally may be more likely to smoke than healthy people. Thus, the estimate of relative risk from Doll and Hill's study may be an underestimate of the true relative risk. The selection of an appropriate control group is fraught with difficulties and is much more difficult than it sounds.

The retrospective nature of the case–control study poses special problems for the measurement of exposure. Study participants are interviewed about characteristics and behaviors that occurred in the past, and some events and characteristics might be difficult to place in time. Moreover, there may be problems with selective recall, especially among the cases, who may be motivated to report exposures that they think might explain their disease. Differences in exposure between cases and controls might stem from this selective recall instead of from any true difference in the exposure.

Strengths and Weaknesses of Case–Control Studies

Strengths

- Efficient design for rare conditions or outcomes;
- Logistically efficient for diseases with long induction or latency periods;
- Can effectively examine several exposures in one study.

Weaknesses

- Susceptible to selection bias;
- Susceptible to recall bias;
- May be difficult to establish that the exposure precedes the outcome;
- Inefficient for studying rare exposures.

Cohort Studies

A *cohort study*—sometimes called a panel study, a follow-up study, or a prospective study—begins with a collection of people who do not have the condition or outcome of interest. This group is then followed over time to discover whether an exposure differentially predicts the outcome. Are the people with the exposure more likely to develop the disease? (Walter, Kamrin, & Katz, 2000). A well-known cohort study is the Nurses' Health Study in which 120,000 nurses were recruited to complete a baseline questionnaire in 1976. Every 2 years, members of this group (or *cohort*) have completed questionnaires that include questions about a wide variety of exposures, diseases, and health-related topics that include smoking, hormone use, diet, and menopausal status. Disease incidence among those with the exposure is subsequently compared with disease incidence in those without the exposure. Data from the Nurses' Health Study have demonstrated, for example, that eating fish more than once a week reduces the risk of coronary heart disease (Hu et al., 2002), while cigarette smoking increases the risk (Willett et al., 1987).

Cohort Study Example

In 1976, a random sample of nearly 20,000 adults living in Copenhagen completed a questionnaire about various health issues including smoking, drinking alcohol, and body weight. The study participants were tracked until 1988, when death certificates were obtained for the more than 2,000 participants who had died. The rate of death from cardiovascular and cerebrovascular disease was 55% lower among those who drank three to five glasses of wine a day compared with nondrinkers. People who drank three to five beers daily were 30% less likely to die from cardiovascular or cerebrovascular disease, but were 20% more likely to die from all causes (Gronbaek et al., 1995).

For exposures that are relatively common (such as smoking, drinking, or using oral contraceptives), investigators may assemble an initial cohort without specifically choosing members based on their exposures. For example, participants in the Nurses' Health Study were enrolled whether or not they were smokers or users of oral contraceptives (two of the exposures of interest for the study). For exposures that are less common, such as exposure to industrial chemicals, investigators may enroll specific groups of people with and without exposure.

A cohort study has a number of strengths. Because cohort members can be selected based on exposure, this design is efficient for studying rare exposures. The prospective nature of the cohort study and the initial selection of people without disease ensure that the exposure precedes the disease, therefore strengthening causal inferences. Of course, these advantages are offset by some disadvantages. The cohort study is an inefficient way to study rare diseases. Even in the Nurses' Health Study, with 120,000 participants, there were simply not enough cases of such rare conditions as liver cancer to study the predictors of this disease.

A cohort study is also subject to attrition, as participants drop out over the course of the study. If this attrition is related to an exposure of interest, then the results can be biased. For example, suppose that in a cohort study of the long-term effects of smoking, people who smoked and developed health problems were more likely to drop out of the study between the initial assessment and the final follow-up. The loss of these participants would result in an estimate of relative risk that was lower than the true value. Moreover, people with and without the exposure at the outset of the study may differ in unknown ways that might not be measured in the study. For example, heavy drinkers or smokers may also have habits that can adversely affect their health, including a poor diet or lack of exercise; these unknown factors, instead of the exposure of interest, may be responsible for different rates of disease in exposed and unexposed cohort members.

As in any study, accurate measurement of exposures is crucial. Studies of alcohol consumption pose particular difficulties. Drinking can be variable over time, making analysis difficult (Jick, Garcia Rodriguez, & Perez-Gutthann, 1998). Drinking patterns include a number of aspects of consumption, including quantity, frequency, and duration, which might be related differently to various outcomes, and ideally the study would seek to measure carefully all these aspects of consumption. In many of the cohort studies that reported the effects of alcohol consumption, however, alcohol was not a major focus of interest in the design of the study, and drinking measures are rudimentary. Measures of general volume, used in many cohort studies, do not reflect important variations in drinking patterns. For example, consuming seven drinks per week might reflect having one drink each evening, or six drinks on a Saturday night and one on Sunday morning, or any number of other patterns. The health outcomes and social consequences of different drinking patterns are not the same.

Strengths and Weaknesses of Cohort Studies

Strengths

- Efficient design for studying rare exposures;
- Ensures that the exposure precedes the outcome.

Weaknesses

- Can be costly and time-consuming;
- Loss of participants during follow-up can affect the comparability of exposed and unexposed groups;
- Inefficient design for rare diseases or conditions;
- Exposed and unexposed groups can differ in unmeasured ways at the outset of the study.

Clinical Trials

A *clinical trial*, also called a randomized controlled trial (RCT) or experimental study, is, like a cohort study, a prospective study in which participants are followed up to determine rates of disease. In a clinical trial, however, the researcher manipulates the exposure: Participants are randomly assigned to discrete groups representing different treatments or interventions. The clinical trial is thus an analogue of a laboratory experiment in which the scientist manipulates the conditions instead of observing naturally occurring exposures. Clearly, an experimenter cannot manipulate many exposures, and the main application of this study design is to test therapeutic interventions. Thus, the focus of this kind of study is not to assess a relationship of a risk factor to an outcome but to test ways to prevent or reduce the outcome.

In alcohol research, clinical trials might be used to test different treatments for alcohol-dependent individuals. *Community trials*, in which communities are assigned to different treatment conditions, are used to test the effects of community-wide interventions on alcohol-related outcomes. For example, in a five-year project in three locations in the U.S. (Holder, 2000; Holder et al., 1997), five interventions were implemented at the community level. These included mobilizing the community to develop organization and support, encouraging responsible beverage service at bars and restaurants, reducing retail availability of alcohol to minors, increasing local enforcement of drinking and driving laws, and using zoning to limit the availability of alcohol by controlling alcohol outlets. In the communities that received the intervention, traffic crashes involving alcohol, assault injuries observed in emergency departments, sales to minors, and self-reported heavy drinking were all reduced.

Choice of Analytic Study Design

The choice of a study design is guided by a number of factors, including cost, time constraints, and the characteristics of the exposures and outcomes of interest. Case–control studies are an appropriate choice for studying rare conditions that would be nearly impossible to study with cohort studies; however, case–control studies are not particularly efficient for examining uncommon exposures. Whereas case–control studies can be used to examine multiple predictors of a single outcome, cohort studies can be used to examine multiple outcomes of the same exposure. Cohort studies are costly and time-consuming, however, and it may take years to collect data on diseases that develop over time.

In alcohol research, we may be concerned mostly with the effects of different drinking patterns on morbidity and mortality in general; thus, we might choose a cohort study to examine the relationship of drinking to several long-term consequences such as cancer, heart disease, cirrhosis, or stroke. If, instead, we want to examine the relationship of drinking to a specific outcome, we might choose a case–control study. Note that many studies of drinking and its consequences use both methods: For example, a recent review of the association of alcohol consumption and breast cancer lists 24 case–control studies and 12 cohort studies (Singletary & Gapstur, 2001).

Some of the consequences of alcohol consumption (e.g., liver cirrhosis) are long-term (chronic) conditions that develop over years; other consequences (e.g., a car accident resulting from driving while intoxicated) are immediate (acute) and represent specific events instead of conditions. Different methods are required to assess acute and chronic consequences. For chronic consequences, either cohort or case–control studies might be used to assess the association of drinking patterns to the outcome. Acute consequences, however, represent specific events that might be associated with single drinking occasions, instead of general drinking patterns. For these events, such as injuries and criminal activity, the method of study chosen should ensure that drinking at the time of the event is assessed. Case–control studies can be used in such circumstances. For example, in a study of alcohol use and accidental falls in Helsinki, Finland, researchers enrolled 313 people who were injured in accidental falls in public places, and then conducted surveys of 626 pedestrians who were walking in the same locations in which the cases were injured. Blood alcohol levels exceeding .05% were detected in 54% of the cases and 13% of the controls, indicating that drinking to that level was associated with a fivefold increase in the risk of injury (Honkanen et al., 1983).

ERRORS AND BIASES IN EPIDEMIOLOGIC RESEARCH

Estimates of risk from observational epidemiologic studies are subject to two kinds of inaccuracies: *random error*, which is the result of chance variation, and systematic error or *bias*. Consider a bathroom scale that reads inaccurately—sometimes a pound or two low, sometimes a pound or two high, with no particular pattern—but that averages the correct weight. The scale is not very precise and exhibits random error. Consider a second scale that measures weight consistently each time, but always measures two pounds high. This scale is precise, but it is biased (distorted) toward overestimating weight. Similarly, consider a case–control study in which people with and without hypertension are interviewed about their past drinking habits. If the interview questions are badly worded so that people have difficulty answering them correctly, random error is introduced into the estimate of relative risk. But if people with hypertension are more likely to recall heavier alcohol consumption as a way of explaining their condition, the relative risk is biased, or distorted: Because the cases and controls responded to the questions differently, the estimated relative risk is higher than it should be.

Although random error results in a lack of precision, bias leads to a systematic distortion of risk estimates in either direction. Three classes of bias include: *selection bias*, resulting from processes by which subjects are selected into the study; *information bias*, resulting from inaccurate measurement; and *confounding*, resulting from the action of risk factors other than the exposure of interest (Grimes & Schulz, 2002; Hennekens & Buring, 1987; Schoenbach & Rosamond, 2000).

Selection Bias

Selection bias occurs when participants in a study are not representative of the population of interest. A well-known example of selection bias occurred in 1948, when polling organizations predicted that Republican Thomas E. Dewey would win the U.S. presidential election over Democrat Harry Truman. Apparently, the pollsters were more likely to interview Republicans than Democrats, resulting in the famous photograph of Truman holding an advance copy of a newspaper with the headline "Dewey Defeats Truman."

Selection bias results from the way in which subjects are selected for a study and can arise in different ways:

• People who volunteer for a study may be different from those who do not volunteer.
• In a cohort study, people who drop out of a study may be different from those who continue.
• In a case–control study, the control group may not be typical of people without the disease.
• In a case–control study, the exposure increases or decreases the likelihood of detecting a case.
• In a case–control study, the exposure has some influence on the selection of controls (the presence of the exposure in the controls will then be different from that in the base population).

The result is that the groups are not comparable to one another and differ in some important way that has nothing to do with the exposure of interest (Grimes & Schulz, 2002). As a result, the measure of association is biased, either upward or downward.

Consider, for example, a cohort study of alcohol consumption and heart disease in which participants are followed up for a number of years. Cohort studies usually lose some participants along the way; this is to be expected. If there is a different rate of dropout in the different groups of the study, however, bias can result. If, in this example, drinkers who became ill with heart disease were more likely to drop out than other participants were, the rate of heart disease for drinkers would be underestimated. The relative risk of heart disease for drinkers vs. nondrinkers would then be biased downward and would be smaller than it should be.

In case–control studies, selection bias is always a potential problem, and careful attention must be paid to selection of both cases and controls. Selection bias in case–control studies occurs when the case and control groups differ in important ways aside from the presence of disease. For example, selection bias occurs if the exposure of interest affects the likelihood that a case will be identified. Several studies (Cherpitel, 1993; Cherpitel et al., 2003) have investigated whether alcohol is associated with injuries by comparing people who arrive at a hospital emergency department with injuries (cases) with those who visit the emergency department for other reasons (controls). An injured person's use of alcohol may influence the decision to seek medical care; an intoxicated person might be more likely to be transported to the hospital if friends or paramedics interpret slurred speech as an indication of brain injury instead of intoxication, or if they fear that otherwise an injured victim might pass out in the street. Drinking victims would then be more likely to show up in the emergency department than would sober victims with similar injuries. Thus, intoxicated victims would be overrepresented among emergency department clients, making it appear as if alcohol increases the risk of injury (Cummings, Koepsell, & Roberts, 2001).

When controls for hospital-based cases are also selected from hospitals, selection bias can occur when both the exposure and the disease influence the likelihood of hospital admission. Continuing with the example of alcohol and injury, controls selected from those who visit the emergency department are likely to be atypical of the base population in terms of alcohol consumption: Drinking is associated with many other health conditions that might lead a person to seek medical care.

Information Bias

Information bias is the result of errors in defining, measuring, or classifying variables of interest. These errors can be the product of inaccurate diagnostic procedures, badly worded questionnaires and interviews, or faulty measurement devices. If these errors are similar for both groups in a study (cases and controls, or exposed and unexposed people), the result is a lack of precision in the estimate of association, but no systematic bias. If the errors are unevenly distributed across study groups, however, they can lead to either inflated or attenuated estimates of association.

One example of information bias is *recall bias*, which occurs when study participants report on their past experiences inaccurately. This form of bias is particularly problematic in case–control studies, in which cases and controls are interviewed about their past histories, including information on the exposure of interest. Because people with a disease may be more motivated to try to understand the causes of their condition, they may be more likely to search their memories rigorously to recall exposures, or even to falsely report some exposure. The result is a measure of association that is stronger than it would be without the bias.

For example, in a case–control study of birth defects and alcohol consumption during pregnancy, mothers who have given birth to an infant with malformations may be more likely to report drinking during pregnancy, either because these malformations produce more thorough recall among these mothers, or because these mothers overreport the drinking in order to explain the outcome. If recall bias is operating, the observed association of drinking and fetal abnormalities will be overestimated. An illustration of the potential impact of recall bias is a comparison of results from case–control studies and cohort studies of the association of oral contraceptives and cancer. Whereas case–control studies demonstrate an association of oral contraceptives and cancer, cohort studies find no association. This discrepancy might be explained with reference to recall bias in the case–control studies, which would tend to inflate the estimated association (Taubes, 1995).

A second way that information bias can operate is through systematic errors in classifying exposure and disease. Researchers might make incorrect diagnoses or make mistakes in determining exposures. Bias occurs when these errors differ among study groups. Suppose, for example, that in a case–control study of alcohol consumption and esophageal cancer, physicians interview the cases in person and the controls are interviewed over the telephone by survey interviewers. Study participants are likely to respond differently to physicians than to telephone interviewers, and might then report their drinking histories differently in the two groups. If the participants are more likely to report truthfully to the physicians but to underreport their drinking to telephone interviewers, then any differences in drinking measures between cases and controls could be caused by the interview method instead of the drinking itself.

Confounding

Confounding refers to the distortion of an association of exposure to the outcome, which is brought about by an extraneous factor (Gerstman, 1998). If we observe an association between an exposure and an outcome, there may be other superfluous factors that are actually "driving" the relationship. Thus, differences in the occurrence of disease are due not to the exposure but to the *confounder,* which is associated with both the exposure and the disease.

Consider the question of whether alcohol consumption increases risk for lung cancer, and suppose that research finds that heavier drinkers are indeed more likely to develop lung cancer. Cigarette smoking confounds this association. Smoking is an independent risk factor for lung cancer, and smoking is associated with drinking (heavier drinkers are more likely to smoke). Thus, heavier drinkers may be more likely to develop lung cancer not because they drink, but because they smoke. The extent of this confounding was evaluated in a case–control study (Zang & Wynder, 2001); the findings showed that when smoking was not taken into account, heavier drinkers were 2.4 times more likely to have lung cancer than were nondrinkers. When the effect of smoking was statistically adjusted, however, alcohol had no effect on lung cancer.

Confounding arises in observational epidemiologic research because of the lack of control over the variables being studied (Coggon, Rose, & Barker, 1997; Schoenbach & Rosamond, 2000). In laboratory research, the scientist can easily alter one variable at a time; for example, an experimental group of rats can be injected with a drug while the control group is injected with a saline solution. Other than the experimental manipulation, the conditions under which the rats live are identical. In the real world, however, exposures and diseases are interrelated in complex ways, and confounding is the bane of the epidemiologist's existence.

Alcohol consumption is an independent risk factor for a number of health conditions, and it is also associated with other exposures, including smoking and diet, as well as sociodemographic characteristics such as gender and age. Thus, any study of the risks or benefits associated with alcohol is subject to potential confounding effects that can obscure the effects of a true cause or can give rise to spurious associations when, in fact, there is no causal relation. Confounding can occur in any kind of analytic design. In ecological studies, discussed earlier in this chapter, populations that show high drinking rates and low rates of heart disease also have other dietary characteristics linked with drinking rates that may explain low levels of heart disease. In cohort studies, the moderate drinking rates that are associated with lower risk may be markers for healthier lifestyles. For example, it has been suggested that wine drinkers tend to be better educated, wealthier, and smoke less than those who prefer other kinds of beverage alcohol (Mortensen, Jensen, Sanders, & Reinisch, 2001).

George Bernard Shaw (1911) offers an excellent description of confounding:

> . . . Comparisons which are really comparisons between two social classes with different standards of nutrition and education are palmed off as comparisons between the results of certain medical treatment and its neglect. Thus it is easy to prove that the wearing of tall hats and the carrying of umbrellas enlarges the chest, prolongs life, and confers comparative immunity from disease; for the statistics show that the classes which use these articles are bigger, healthier, and live longer than the class which never dreams of possessing such things. It does not take much perspicacity to see that what really makes this difference is not the tall hat and the umbrella, but the wealth and nourishment of which they are

evidence, and that a gold watch or membership of a club in Pall Mall might be proved in the same way to have the like sovereign virtues. A university degree, a daily bath, the owning of thirty pairs of trousers, a knowledge of Wagner's music, a pew in church, anything, in short, that implies more means and better nurture than the mass of laborers enjoy, can be statistically palmed off as a magic-spell conferring all sorts of privileges (p. 1xiv).

Errors and biases are inevitable in epidemiologic research, but their importance is a matter of interpretation. Designing studies to minimize error and bias takes thought, care, and good planning, all of which are usually in good supply among epidemiologists. Although assessment of bias is part of interpreting the results of a study, sometimes criticisms of bias are invoked indiscriminately to question conclusions (Jick, Garcia Rodriguez, & Perez-Gutthann, 1998). The presence of bias in a study does not mean that it is scientifically unacceptable and should be disregarded (Coggon, Rose, & Barker, 1997).

INTERPRETING EPIDEMIOLOGIC RESEARCH: THE ROLE OF UNCERTAINTY

"There is something fascinating about science. One gets such wholesale returns of conjecture out of such a trifling investment of fact."

Mark Twain, 1883

The increasing amount of media attention to health-related research has highlighted an aspect of scientific research that is little understood: the role of uncertainty. Epidemiologists, in particular, have gotten a bad reputation. For example, an article in *Scientific American* said that although "epidemiologists are the unsung heroes of medicine . . . epidemiologists drive us crazy" (Mirsky, 2000). The author complains that his head spins when confronted with conflicting findings that report drinking is good for us (heart-wise) but bad for us (increasing risky behavior). More thoughtful treatments of the issue of uncertainty have appeared in *Science* and the *New England Journal of Medicine.* In *Science,* science writer Gary Taubes noted that "The news about health risks comes thick and fast these days, and it seems almost constitutionally contradictory" (Taubes, 1995, p. 164) before going on to interview several prominent epidemiologists about the state of the discipline. Marcia Angell, the editor of the *New England Journal of Medicine,* noted that "health-conscious Americans increasingly find themselves beset by contradictory advice. No sooner do they learn the results of one research study than they hear of one with the opposite message" (Angell & Kassirer, 1994, p. 189). Media reports highlight the controversies: "Why can't researchers get it straight the first time?" (Angell & Kassirer, 1994, p. 189).

In Angell's view, the problem lies not with the research but with the way it is interpreted for the public. Science is not a set of facts or pieces of received wisdom, but a process—one that is not always linear. Single studies represent steps in the process, but actually cannot provide what people want: simple guidelines to follow to improve their health. Although such guidelines might emerge through repeated research, often the public and the media don't want to wait for the process to work.

Looking at research studies as part of the scientific process, we see that new studies should be viewed not as end points but as discussions among scientists—dialogues "characterized by cycles of revisions, conjectures, assertions, and contradictions" (International Food Information Council, 2000). Single studies, which cannot stand alone as definitive, provide parts of an accumulated body of evidence that points in the same direction.

Contradictory research findings stem from several characteristics of the scientific process:

- Hypotheses about cause and effect cannot be proven with the scientific method. The best that can be said is that research *supports* a hypothesis. The results of a study could always be a fluke or the result of chance, even if the probability of that is small.
- Except for census taking, which attempts to gather data from every member of a population, studies use samples of people selected from the population of interest. The sampling procedure can introduce uncertainty into the results, given that any sample will differ—even if only slightly—from the general population. Moreover, different samples will differ from one another (Walter, Kamrin, & Katz, 2000). For example, if the population prevalence of a particular condition is 10%, one sample might have 9% prevalence and another 15%, merely due to chance, making the two samples look different when the population is really the same (Walter et al., 2000).
- Methods and studies differ from each another in many ways (Walter et al., 2000). As we have discussed, different study designs have differing sources of error and bias, and the estimates of risk calculated from these studies are imprecise. The degree of precision of a study varies with its methodology and with the rarity of the condition being examined.
- When associations between exposure and disease are relatively weak, studies may show contradictory results. Taubes (1995) notes that in the past 50 years, epidemiology has identified the most conspicuous health risks, including smoking, which is very strongly related to lung cancer. Currently, scientists are looking for risk factors with weaker and subtler links between diseases and lifestyles or environmental causes. These subtle risks can affect a large segment of the population, which gives them huge impact; however, the limitations of epidemiology mean that these

associations are difficult to interpret. As epidemiologist Michael Thun put it, "With epidemiology you can tell a little thing from a big thing. What's very hard to do is to tell a little thing from nothing at all" (Taubes, 1995, p. 164).

• Uncertainty and inconsistency can result from the search for multiple determinants of health outcomes, which are the product of biological, environmental, societal, and behavioral factors. Investigating these multiple determinants, many of which cannot be easily measured, is complex, and frequently equivocal findings are the result (Sly, 1996).

• Results from studies of different populations may be very different. For example, research on the association of alcohol consumption and liver damage have found important differences in men and women: Women develop alcohol-induced liver disease over a shorter period of time and after consuming less alcohol (Gavaler & Arria, 1995; Tuyns & Pequignot, 1984).

• Despite the best efforts of scientists, some studies are simply poorly designed and implemented. These limitations can increase apparent inconsistencies between studies (Sly, 1996).

Contradictory study findings can be overemphasized by journalists because of the way these findings are presented to readers:

• Different journalists may present the same study findings in different ways (Dunwoody, 1999). For example, the two local newspapers in Seattle, Washington, both reported on a study of the effects of antioxidants, cholesterol-lowering drugs called statins, and their combination on cholesterol levels (Brown et al., 2001). Patients who took statins (in combination with niacin) showed improved cholesterol levels and lower risk of heart attack after 3 years; among patients who took antioxidants, cholesterol levels were unchanged and risk of heart attack was increased compared with the placebo condition. These findings were presented quite differently in the two newspapers: The *Seattle Times* emphasized the beneficial effects of statins with a headline that read: "Heart Trouble Reduced in Study: Drug–Niacin Mix May Reverse Disease" (King, 2001). The *Seattle Post-Intelligencer* focused on the poor showing of antioxidants in an article headlined: "Anti-oxidants May Hinder Some Drugs" (Haney, 2001).

• An unstated "balance norm" encourages journalists to give equal space to competing points of view, even when the two sides are not equally legitimate. This focus on "dueling experts," with equal weight given to majority and fringe scientific views and no discussion of the reasons for the discrepancies, can make issues appear more uncertain than they really are (Dunwoody, 1999; Stocking, 1999).

• Journalists tend to present studies in isolation, instead of in the context of other research. A writer may spotlight one study that showed a positive association of an exposure and disease, without reference to several studies showing no association. For example, the *New York Times* reported that a new study found that having an abortion was associated with a 50% increase in breast cancer. Although the article noted that 40 previous studies had found no association of abortion to breast cancer, the headline read: "New Study Links Abortions and Increase in Breast Cancer Risk" (Mann, 1995). (In defense of journalists, some of this emphasis comes from press releases from scientific and medical journals that tout new findings.)

Journalists are sometimes accused of making research findings sound more certain than they really are. Journalistic accounts tend to have fewer caveats than the scientific reports upon which they are based; they also tend to lack historical context and discussion of previous research on the topic (Stocking, 1999). "While scientists are socialized to qualify their findings, journalists often see qualification as protective colouration. Furthermore, readability in the eyes of a journalist may be over-simplification to a scientist" (Nelkin, 1996).

At the same time, by presenting inconsistent research findings without explanation or discussion of potential reasons for the contradictions, journalists, at times, make scientific claims appear more uncertain than most scientists believe them to be (Mirsky, 2000; Stocking, 1999). The role of the media is discussed in detail in Chapter 4, which addresses the general concept of communicating risks.

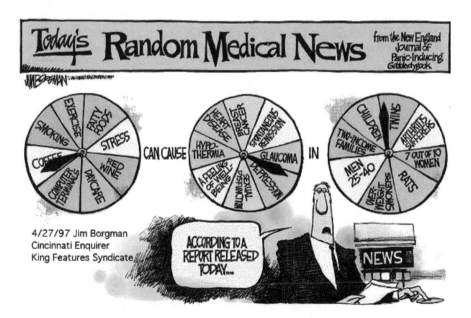

Copyright 1997. Reprinted with special permission of King Features Syndicate.

SUMMARY

In today's world, chronic diseases, such as heart disease and cancer, are of greater public health importance than the infectious diseases that were the great killers of a century ago. The health and lifestyle factors that may predispose us to these chronic diseases are complex and interrelated (Walter et al., 2000), a far cry from the single germs that were discovered and nearly eradicated by previous generations of scientists. Despite its limitations, epidemiologic research is the best available approach for studying these increasingly complex phenomena (Trichopoulos, 1995).

Many epidemiologists believe that people are more impressed with the overall record of epidemiology than worried about the controversies it engenders (Morabia, 2001). Modern-day epidemiology has provided the knowledge we now have about the prevention of chronic disease by discovering and investigating associations between smoking and lung cancer, sun exposure and skin cancer, and obesity and morbidity. Moreover, epidemiologic research has been able to provide some reassurance about suspected risk factors, demonstrating that saccharin use is not related to increased risk of bladder cancer and that oral contraceptives do not increase the risk of cancer (Morabia, 2001; Willett et al., 1995).

Although individual studies will always be uncertain, epidemiology depends on the replication and confirmation of research findings; repeated studies and the preponderance of evidence can ultimately tip the balance in favor of an explanation (Walter et al., 2000). Understanding the process of science can help the consumer of scientific research reserve judgment about individual studies without "succumbing to antiscientific nihilism" (Angell & Kassirer, 1994, p.190).

REFERENCES

American Cancer Society. (2001). Alcohol intake tied to breast cancer risk. Retrieved October 7, 2003, from http://www.cancer.org.

Angell, M., & Kassirer, J. P. (1994). Clinical research—What should the public believe? *New England Journal of Medicine, 331*(3), 189–190.

Armstrong, B., & Doll, R. (1975). Environmental factors and cancer incidence and mortality in different countries, with special reference to dietary practices. *International Journal of Cancer, 15*(4), 617–631.

Bonner, R., & Fessenden, F. (2000, September 22). States with no death penalty share lower homicide rates. *New York Times*, pp. 1, 19.

Brown, B. G., Zhao, X. Q., Chait, A., Fisher, L. D., Cheung, M. C., Morse, J. S., et al. (2001). Simvastatin and niacin, antioxidant vitamins, or the combination for the prevention of coronary disease. *New England Journal of Medicine, 345*(22), 1583–1592.

Cady, L. D., Bischoff, D. P., O'Connell, E. R., Thomas, P. C., & Allan, J. H. (1979). Strength and fitness and subsequent back injuries in firefighters. *Journal of Occupational Medicine, 21*(4), 269–272.

Cherpitel, C. J. (1993). Alcohol and injuries: A review of international emergency room studies. *Addiction, 88*(7), 923–937.

Cherpitel, C. J., Bond, J., Ye, Y., Borges, G., Macdonald, S., & Giesbrecht, N. (2003). A cross-national meta-analysis of alcohol and injury: Data from the Emergency Room Collaborative Alcohol Analysis Project (ERCAAP). *Addiction, 98*(9), 1277–1286.

Coggon, D., Rose, G., & Barker, D. J. P. (1997). *Epidemiology for the uninitiated.* Retrieved from http://bmj.com/epidem.

Cohen, L. E., & Felson, M. (1979). Social change and crime rate trends: A routine activities approach. *American Sociological Review, 44,* 588–607.

Collins, J. J. (1993). Drinking and violence: An individual offender focus. In S. E. Martin (Ed.), *Alcohol and interpersonal violence: Fostering multidisciplinary perspectives* (Vol. NIAAA, Research Monograph No. 24, NIH Pub 93-3496, pp. 221–235). Rockville, MD: U.S. Department of Health and Human Services.

Collins, J. J., & Messerschmidt, P. M. (1993). Epidemiology of alcohol-related violence. Special Issue: Alcohol, aggression, and injury. *Alcohol Health & Research World, 17*(2), 93–100.

Cummings, P., & Weiss, N. S. (1998). Case series and exposure series: The role of studies without controls in providing information about the etiology of injury or disease. *Injury Prevention, 4*(1), 54–57.

Cummings, P., Koepsell, T. D., & Roberts, I. (2001). Case-control studies in injury research. In F. P. Rivara, P. Cummings, T. D. Koepsell, D. C. Grossman, & R. V. Maier (Eds.), *Injury control: A guide to research and program evaluation* (pp. 139–156). New York: Cambridge University Press.

Divers Alert Network. (2003). *Report on decompression illness, diving fatalities and Project Dive Exploration.* Durham, NC: Divers Alert Network.

Doll, R., & Hill, A. B. (1950). Smoking and carcinoma of the lung: Preliminary report. *British Medical Journal, 2,* 739–748.

Dunwoody, S. (1999). Scientists, journalists, and the meaning of uncertainty. In S. M. Friedman, S. Dunwoody, & C. L. Rogers (Eds.), *Communicating uncertainty: Media coverage of new and controversial science* (pp. 59–79). Mahwah, NJ: Lawrence Erlbaum.

Eagan, T. M., Gulsvik, A., Eide, G. E., & Bakke, P. S. (2002). Occupational airborne exposure and the incidence of respiratory symptoms and asthma. *American Journal of Respiratory and Critical Care Medicine, 166*(7), 933–938.

Evans, C. M. (1986). Alcohol and violence: Problems relating to methodology, statistics and causation. In P. F. Brain (Ed.), *Alcohol and aggression* (pp. 138–160). London: Croom Helm.

Gavaler, J. S., & Arria, A. M. (1995). Increased susceptibility of women to alcoholic liver disease: Artifactual or real? In P. Hall (Ed.), *Alcoholic liver disease: Pathology and pathogenesis (2nd Ed.)* (pp. 123–133). London: Edward Arnold.

Gerstman, B. B. (1998). *Epidemiology kept simple.* New York: John Wiley.

Goodwin, D. W., Crane, J. B., & Guze, S. B. (1971). Felons who drink: An eight-year follow-up. *Quarterly Journal of Studies on Alcohol, 32,* 136–147.

Gottlieb, M. S., Schanker, H. M., Fan, P. T., Saxon, A., Weisman, J. D., & Pozalski, I. (1981). Pneumocystis pneumonia—Los Angeles. *Morbidity and Mortality Weekly Report, 30*(21), 1–3.

Graham, K., Schmidt, G., & Gillis, K. (1996). Circumstances when drinking leads to aggression: An overview of research findings. *Contemporary Drug Problems, 23*(3), 493–558.

Greenberg, B. (1999, November 18). An alcoholic drink each week may reduce stroke risk. *Seattle Times* (Associated Press).

Greenfeld, L. A. (1998). *Alcohol and crime: An analysis of national data on the prevalence of alcohol involvement in crime*. Washington, DC: Bureau of Justice Statistics.

Grimes, D. A., & Schulz, K. F. (2002). Bias and causal associations in observational research. *Lancet, 359*(9302), 248–252.

Gronbaek, M., Deis, A., Sorensen, T. I., Becker, U., Schnohr, P., & Jensen, G. (1995). Mortality associated with moderate intakes of wine, beer, or spirits. *British Medical Journal, 310*(6988), 1165–1169.

Haney, D. Q. (2001, November 29). Anti-oxidants may hinder some drugs. *Seattle Post-Intelligencer* (Associated Press).

Hennekens, C. H., & Buring, J. E. (1987). *Epidemiology in medicine*. Boston: Little, Brown.

Holder, H. D. (2000). Community prevention of alcohol problems. *Addictive Behaviors, 25*(6), 843–859.

Holder, H. D., Saltz, R. F., Grube, J. W., Voas, R. B., Gruenewald, P. J., & Treno, A. J. (1997). A community prevention trial to reduce alcohol-involved accidental injury and death: overview. *Addiction, 92*, S155–S171.

Honkanen, R., Ertama, L., Kuosmanen, P., Linnoila, M., Alha, A., & Visuri, T. (1983). The role of alcohol in accidental falls. *Journal of Studies on Alcohol, 44*(2), 231–245.

Hu, F. B., Bronner, L., Willett, W. C., Stampfer, M. J., Rexrode, K. M., Albert, C. M., et al. (2002). Fish and omega-3 fatty acid intake and risk of coronary heart disease in women. *Journal of the American Medical Association, 287*(14), 1815–1821.

International Food Information Council (IFIC). (2000). IFIC Review: How to understand and interpret food and health-related scientific studies. Retrieved from http://ific.org.

Jick, H., Garcia Rodriguez, L. A., & Perez-Gutthann, S. (1998). Principles of epidemiological research on adverse and beneficial drug effects. *Lancet, 352*(9142), 1767–1770.

Johnson, T. (1998). Shattuck lecture—Medicine and the media. *New England Journal of Medicine, 339*(2), 87–92.

Kalish, C. (1983). *Prisoners and alcohol*. Washington, DC: U.S. Department of Justice, Bureau of Justice Statistics.

Kaposi's sarcoma and *Pneumocystis* pneumonia among homosexual men—New York City and California (1981). *Morbidity and Mortality Weekly Report, 30*(25), 305–308.

Kim, K., Uchiyama, M., Okawa, M., Doi, Y., Oida, T., Minowa, M., et al. (1999). Lifestyles and sleep disorders among the Japanese adult population. *Psychiatry and Clinical Neurosciences, 53*(2), 269–270.

King, W. (2001, November 29). Heart trouble reduced in study: Drug-niacin mix may reverse disease. *Seattle Times*.

Kleinbaum, D. G., Kupper, L. L., & Morgenstern, H. (1982). *Epidemiologic research: Principles and quantitative methods*. New York: Van Nostrand Reinhold.

Ladouceur, P., & Temple, M. (1985). Substance use among rapists: A comparison with other serious felons. *Crime and Delinquency, 31*(2), 269–294.

Last, J. M. (2001). *A dictionary of epidemiology*. Oxford: Oxford University Press.

Lewin, T. (2001, December 17). Conflicting breast cancer studies creating unsettling uncertainties. *New York Times*, p. 1.

Li, G., Baker, S. P., Smialek, J. E., & Soderstrom, C. A. (2001). Use of alcohol as a risk factor for bicycling injury. *Journal of the American Medical Association, 285*(7), 893–896.

Lipsey, M. W., Wilson, D. B., Cohen, M. A., & Derzon, J. H. (1997). Is there a causal relationship between alcohol use and violence? A synthesis of evidence. In M. Galanter (Ed.), *Recent developments in alcoholism* (Vol. 13: *Alcohol and violence*, pp. 245–282). New York: Plenum Press.

Maier, S. E., & West, J. R. (2001). Drinking patterns and alcohol-related birth defects. *Alcohol Research and Health, 25*(3), 168–174.

Mann, C. C. (1995). Press coverage: Leaving out the big picture. *Science, 269*(5221), 166.

Mirsky, S. (2000). Alcohol, tobacco and soy alarms. *Scientific American, 283*(1), 112.

Morabia, A. (2001). The essential tension between absolute and relative causality. *American Journal of Public Health, 91*(3), 355–357.

Mortensen, E. L., Jensen, H. H., Sanders, S. A., & Reinisch, J. M. (2001). Better psychological functioning and higher social status may largely explain the apparent health benefits of wine: a study of wine and beer drinking in young Danish adults. *Archives of Internal Medicine, 161*(15), 1844–1848.

National Highway Traffic Safety Administration. (2001). *Traffic safety facts 2001* (No. DOT HS 809 476).

National Institute on Alcohol Abuse and Alcoholism. (1993). Alcohol and cancer. *Alcohol Alert, 21.*

National Institute on Alcohol Abuse and Alcoholism. (1999). Alcohol and coronary heart disease. *Alcohol Alert, 45.*

Nelkin, D. (1995). *Selling science: How the press covers science and technology.* New York: W. H. Freeman.

Nelkin, D. (1996). An uneasy relationship: The tensions between medicine and the media. *Lancet, 347*(9015), 1600–1603.

Parker, R. N., & Cartmill, R. S. (1998). Alcohol and homicide in the United States 1934–1995—or one reason why U.S. rates of violence may be going down. *Journal of Criminal Law and Criminology, 88*(4), 1369–1398.

Parker, R. N., & Rebhun, L.-A. (1995). *Alcohol and homicide: A deadly combination of two American traditions.* Albany, NY: State University of New York Press.

Pittman, D. J., & Gordon, C. W. (1958). Criminal careers of the chronic police case inebriate. *Quarterly Journal of Studies on Alcohol, 19,* 255–268.

Pott, P. (1778). *The chirurgical works of Percivall Pott, FRS.* Dublin: James Williams.

Ries, L. A. G., Eisner, M. P., Kosary, C. L., Hankey, B. F., Miller, B. A., Clegg, L., et al. (Eds.). (2003). *SEER cancer statistics review, 1975–2000* (Vol. 2003). Bethesda, MD: National Cancer Institute.

Rimm, E. B., Klatsky, A., Grobbee, D., & Stampfer, M. J. (1996). Review of moderate alcohol consumption and reduced risk of coronary heart disease: Is the effect due to beer, wine, or spirits? *British Medical Journal, 312*(7033), 731–736.

Rose, G. (1985). Sick individuals and sick populations. *International Journal of Epidemiology, 14*(1), 32–38.

Ross, E. (2002, January 25). Drink or three a day deters dementia, study concludes. *Seattle Times* (Associated Press).

Schoenbach, V. J., & Rosamond, W. D. (2000). *Fundamentals of epidemiology.* Chapel Hill, NC: Department of Epidemiology, University of North Carolina.

Shaw, G. B. (1911). *The doctor's dilemma: Preface on doctors.* New York: Brentano's.

Singletary, K. W., & Gapstur, S. M. (2001). Alcohol and breast cancer: Review of epidemiologic and experimental evidence and potential mechanisms. *Journal of the American Medical Association, 286*(17), 2143–2151.

Sly, T. (1996). Sources of epidemiological equivocacy. *Risk: Health, Safety & Environment, 7,* 1.

Stocking, S. H. (1999). How journalists deal with scientific uncertainty. In S. M. Friedman, S. Dunwoody, & C. L. Rogers (Eds.), *Communicating uncertainty: Media coverage of new and controversial science* (pp. 23–41). Mahwah, NJ: Lawrence Erlbaum.

Taubes, G. (1995). Epidemiology faces its limits. *Science, 269*(5221), 164–169.

Trichopoulos, D. (1995). The discipline of epidemiology. *Science, 269*(5229), 1326.

Tuyns, A. J., & Pequignot, G. (1984). Greater risk of ascitic cirrhosis in females in relation to alcohol consumption. *International Journal of Epidemiology, 13*(1), 53–57.

Walter, M. L., Kamrin, M. A., & Katz, D. (2000). *Reporting on risk.* Retrieved from http://www.facsnet.org/tools/ref_tutor/risk/index.php3.

White, H. R. (1997). Longitudinal perspective on alcohol use and aggression during adolescence. In M. Galanter (Ed.), *Recent developments in alcoholism* (Vol. 13: *Alcohol and violence,* pp. 81–103). New York: Plenum Press.

Willett, W., Greenland, S., MacMahon, B., Trichopoulos, D., Rothman, K., Thomas, D., et al. (1995). The discipline of epidemiology. *Science, 269*(5229), 1325–1326.

Willett, W. C., Green, A., Stampfer, M. J., Speizer, F. E., Colditz, G. A., Rosner, B., et al. (1987). Relative and absolute excess risks of coronary heart disease among women who smoke cigarettes. *New England Journal of Medicine, 317*(21), 1303–1309.

Yokokawa, Y., Ohta, S., Hou, J., Zhang, X. L., Li, S. S., Ping, Y. M., et al. (1999). Ecological study on the risks of esophageal cancer in Ci-Xian, China: The importance of nutritional status and the use of well water. *International Journal of Cancer, 83*(5), 620–624.

Zang, E. A., & Wynder, E. L. (2001). Reevaluation of the confounding effect of cigarette smoking on the relationship between alcohol use and lung cancer risk, with larynx cancer used as a positive control. *Preventive Medicine, 32*(4), 359–370.

Chapter 4

Well-Chosen Words:
Telling the Story of Risk

"If a little knowledge is dangerous, where is a man who has so much as to be out of danger?"

Thomas Henry Huxley (1825–1895)

The latter part of the 20th century witnessed a dramatic expansion in global communication and information exchange. Advances in electronic technology, in particular, have opened the doors to almost instantaneous access to information. Yet, these advances have also opened a Pandora's box of potential pitfalls of misinformation.

The abundance of facts, figures, truths, and half-truths is a reflection of the great strides made in technology and medicine in recent history. As a result, meeting the needs of our daily lives has become, on balance, easier and more convenient; however, the ready accessibility of information has also raised the bar for the skills necessary to navigate safely through what is presented to us. Increasingly, understanding what we are being told appears to require special skills. When dealing with risk information, gauging what requires a response on our part and what does not has become more difficult. We may be unable to fully understand the information before us and to differentiate between risks worth worrying about and those we can reasonably accept or even disregard.

For those of us on the receiving end of risk information, the question becomes how to make sense of what we are told, how to distinguish fact from fiction, and, once we have done so, how to make it applicable to our own lives and value systems. For those in the business of providing such information, the question is how to convey it accurately, evenhandedly, and in a comprehensible fashion—or, whether evenhandedness factors into the equation at all.

As other chapters in this book have attempted to illustrate, how we interpret and deal with risk reflects a complex interplay between our perception of the world around us, our individual value systems, and the cultural prism we apply. These factors play a particularly key role in addressing the relationship between alcohol and risk. This chapter explores the mechanics of risk communication—who is responsible for providing it and how this information is constructed, packaged, and conveyed.

THE COMPLEXITIES OF COMMUNICATING RISKS

For all practical purposes, risk communication can be viewed as any portrayal of danger, whether potential, imminent, or existing, that could place us at peril. Such information may be presented in many forms: as an account of public health concerns, natural disasters, toxic spills or terrorism; as depictions of physical or mental illness; or in any number of other guises. We may read about risk in the print media, see it on television, on billboards, or in film productions. We may hear about it from the health professionals we see or from the government sources that have our attention. We may also receive such information through less formal channels: around the dinner table with friends and family or from colleagues at the office.

The main function of risk communication is to provide the tools that help inform the choices and decisions we make. A hazardous situation becomes meaningful only when we can understand how its consequences relate to us and are able to weigh potential harms against potential benefits. Optimally, risk communication lays out possible alternatives, alerts us to uncertainties, and offers appropriate responses for managing the hazards that are relevant within the context of our lives and everyday experiences. In practice, this standard for risk communication may not necessarily be attainable; yet it is what most of us expect—a simple answer to our worries about how good or bad something is for us as individuals.

In most cultures, alcohol beverages have been consumed since the beginning of recorded history, and possibly longer in many cultures. The immediate effects of alcohol consumption are well known to all who drink and familiar to those who don't. These effects range from the pleasure and well-being associated with moderate and sociable consumption to the physical aftermath of excessive drinking and many of its social and health consequences.

Information about alcohol is abundant and readily available; it has been studied from all possible angles—biomedical, sociological, psychological, political, economic—and the risks associated with certain patterns of drinking and related activities have been well documented (Grant & Litvak, 1998).

In many ways, communicating risk information about alcohol does not differ significantly from communicating information on any number of health issues. What sets risk communication in the alcohol field apart is the charged nature of this particular debate. Everyone has an opinion about alcohol and where (or whether) it fits into society. For some, consuming alcohol is unacceptable, morally wrong, dangerous, and to be avoided at all costs. For others, it is one of life's pleasures, to be enjoyed in moderation, just like fine food or good music. For still others, alcohol dependence and a history of alcohol abuse represent a constant and intensely personal battle.

It has been contended that for most people, most of the time, alcohol consumption is not likely to lead to adverse social or physiological consequences, as long as it is moderate and appropriate for the occasion (Grant & Litvak, 1998). In fact, most of us who drink do so because we enjoy it and are likely to experience few problems. With information about the effects of alcohol prominently featured in daily newspapers and on television, and with warning labels appearing on containers of beer, wine, and distilled spirits in a number of countries around the world, we ask ourselves: How much of this information actually concerns us as individuals? How will drinking affect us directly? How much can we safely drink? What are the issues about which we should be worrying? And, most important, how does the information we are given relate to our lifestyles and to our daily experiences?

Translating Risk Information

Delivering the results of scientific inquiry to the public is a challenging proposition. The first obstacle is that science follows its own rules, and its language is often hard, clinical, and based on probabilities and population averages (see Chapter 3). To the risk expert, a death may be just a death, a figure to include with other mortality data. To those who have lost a loved one, a death is not just a statistic. Risk is closely tied to intuition (i.e., the feeling that something may or may not be safe) and to the belief that personal consequences do matter. Coping with risk is an intensely personal and visceral experience. Some of these facets of risk have been explored more fully in the discussion on how we perceive risk (see Chapter 1).

How we receive and react to information about risk depends to a large extent on how it is packaged. We are likely to react more strongly to information presented to us as immediate and tangible outcomes (e.g., airbags in cars or smoke alarms in buildings) than to discussions of long-term outcomes, some of which may take many years to manifest themselves (e.g., harm resulting from exposure to the sun or smoking).

It is not surprising, therefore, that communications relating to the immediate risks associated with alcohol abuse and with reckless drinking resonate well with the public. Lives lost in traffic accidents because of drunk driving are tangible and highly visible. We instinctively react to them in an emotional way, and it is easy to rally around public measures aimed at preventing them. On the other hand, it is perhaps more difficult to fully appreciate the less immediate risks of alcohol abuse, such as the risk of developing liver cirrhosis because of heavy drinking. Both types of risk are real, but the consequences of one remain invisible and thus often difficult to grasp.

Another obstacle to the easy transfer of scientific information in general and risk information in particular involves the conclusions that can be drawn from a particular situation. Whereas scientists may hesitate about generalizing cause and effect unless the preponderance of the evidence compels them to do so, the public is much more eager to generalize and often needs strong proof *against* making such a link.

In light of the divergence between the spheres of "risk speak" and common language, how does accurate information about risks ever trickle down the knowledge chain? Can risks, whether related to alcohol consumption or any other aspect of life, be communicated in a way that allows us to understand what the numbers mean and why they are relevant to us? And how do we know whom to believe and how to distinguish fact from fiction?

Effective communication about risks combines the rigor of science with comprehensible explanations of the findings. This rule holds true regardless of whether the risks are in the field of health, technology, or any other realm. Good risk communication means expressing complex ideas simply, making them accessible to a wide audience. It depicts the facts accurately and in a way that is pertinent to the issue and, equally important, to the audiences at hand.

Perhaps the most important measure of good risk communication is that it offers a balanced and representative view of the current state of knowledge about a particular topic. Such evenhandedness is crucial because uncertainty and disagreement always exist in scientific analysis. Good risk communication should reflect both mainstream and alternative points of view. In effect, good risk communication seeks to break down the barriers between the spheres of scientific analysis and intuition, facilitating the exchange of information and furthering understanding.

Trusting Sources

When presented with risk information, we must decide whether the information and its source are reliable. Indeed, belief in the integrity of the source is arguably the most critical factor in our reaction to risk information. The source, perhaps more than the actual substance of what we are told, may be the pivotal element in risk communication (Johnson & Slovic, 1994). The degree of trust we are willing to place in the source is crucial to whether we accept the information presented to us.

The decision about whom to trust often reflects our own personal views about authority and whether or not we are inclined to question it, as well as our personal values and priorities. Generally, when it comes to risks, we often have no choice but to place our trust in those who can provide us with facts or those whom we perceive to be concerned with our well-being. These are the "experts" found in government and educational institutions, among health workers and scientists, and in consumer organizations.

In the alcohol field, the experts are the researchers who study the biomedical and social effects of drinking on individuals and society. They are the government sources responsible for providing public information on drinking limits, giving us health advice, and informing us about responsible drinking and prevention of abuse. They are also the medical professionals to whom we turn for guidance because they have experience in the treatment and care of those at risk. The intermediaries through which these experts communicate are those who distill and synthesize the available research and help translate the information into a format that is more easily understood.

Just who belongs to the ranks of experts and authority figures depends on our perception of their knowledge of a particular field and on their general stature in society. Scientists are seen as falling squarely into the group regarded as having expert knowledge and a high degree of integrity, a perception that appears to cut across cultures and is ingrained in the public's mind at an early age. They are considered competent, rigorous, and precise. We regard scientists and the work they do as highly moral and humanitarian, adding to the overall view that we should trust them (Delacôte, 1987).

Another group, however, is high on the trust scale and is comprised of individuals without specialized knowledge or expertise. They are other credible, although not necessarily expert sources: friends, family, or others whom we trust implicitly and in whose hands we are willing to place our safety. In fact, we may trust them more than the "experts" on certain issues (e.g., health care) because they share common concerns (Kaiser Family Foundation & Agency for Healthcare Research and Quality, 1996). Trusted sources also include those whom we believe to possess reliable information about certain risks. We are also more likely to believe what we are told if it is familiar to us and corresponds with our own knowledge and experience of the world.

Much work has been done to disentangle the knotty question of why we choose to trust some sources but not others. It is clear that trust is highly subjective and, at least in theory, boils down to a few basic elements: credibility, integrity, and dependability. How we perceive each of these elements and how important each is to us depends greatly on our personal views and values, as discussed in Chapter 1 on risk perception and Chapter 2 on the role of culture.

Credibility hinges upon whether the claim being made about risk appears to be plausible and whether the source has the necessary expertise, technical sophistication, and detailed knowledge to provide us with accurate information. Do we believe that those who convey information to us are honest and can be trusted?

The trustworthiness test applies as much to individuals as it does to institutions, some of which also fit into the "expert" category. One need only think of government agencies, intergovernmental organizations, nongovernmental bodies, and institutions within the private sector that possess particular expertise and part of whose job it is to communicate information on risk. Entities such as the World Bank, the World Health Organization (WHO), and other United Nations agencies are considered as having (often implicitly) expert stature within their respective fields. By virtue of who they are and what their mandate is, these agencies are relied upon to provide information that is presumed to be accurate, complete, free from bias, and delivered with the public good in mind.

Whether institutions are able to pass the test of credibility, integrity, and dependability has been debated (Borchelt, 2001). Some have argued that within institutions, credibility typically declines as one moves up the hierarchical ladder. Those occupying its lower rungs tend to be there because of their actual expertise, while those at the top of the pyramid, especially within government and other decision-making bodies, may be there for other reasons. Heads of government agencies are commonly political appointees instead of specialists in a given area. Thus, persons who are less credible (by the definitions used here) may, at times, end up telling the story of risk.

As far as the public is concerned, institutions often violate the integrity criterion. Governments appear to evoke a level of public trust so low that they have been reported to rank just above the tabloid press (Frewer, Howard, Hedderley, & Sheperd, 1996, 1998). In general, technology issues appear to be the focus of the public's distrust of government sources, with issues of public health not far behind. To a large extent, this may be the result of past experiences where public health and safety were grossly mishandled by government authorities. The downplaying of the mad cow disease outbreak by the government of the United Kingdom in the 1990s, for instance, or the Chinese government's inertia in the face of the SARS epidemic in 2003 are two such examples. Whether an institution's view of what is involved in protecting the well-being of the public is the same as the public's definition is also a matter of concern (Langford, Marris, & O'Riordan, 1999), as is the fundamental question of whether the public has an inherent right to all the available information, regardless of consequences.

The private sector also typically fares poorly on the scale of public trust when it comes to risk information, but for very different reasons. Where governments are viewed as lacking accountability, the opposite is true for the private sector. Industry sources are generally held accountable for their handling of risk or the dissemination of risk information. As a result, the notion is that this accountability is likely to influence the information that industries choose to communicate and the channels they use to convey their message. Thus, the motives of private-sector sources are often seen as self-serving, largely because of their efforts to avoid being held responsible.

The beverage alcohol industry, like most other industries, has been faced with this criticism. The consequences of heavy and reckless drinking, both health-related and social, are common knowledge. Since the first sips of alcohol were taken by humans, it has been clear that alcohol is a substance, which, when misused, may result in adverse outcomes. The beverage alcohol industry is frequently criticized, however, for not expending sufficient effort to communicate reminders of the potential risks associated with certain patterns of drinking, but communicating alcohol risks is a less straightforward process than that for many other products. In addition to the "common knowledge" issue, certain patterns of alcohol consumption are associated with health and social benefits for some drinkers, and drinking is closely ingrained in many cultures and settings (Heath, 1995, 2000, 2001). The type of information that needs to be communicated and the way it should be formulated is therefore a matter of some contention.

Because corporate interests are perceived as largely driven by balance sheets and the bottom line, attempts made by the alcohol industry to bring both the positive and problematic aspects of its product to the attention of the public are often regarded with skepticism. It is important, however, not to allow the source of information to unduly color the merits of the information itself and to influence how we receive it. The issue is addressed in greater depth in Chapter 6, but it is worth mentioning here that responsible corporate citizenship has been an increasing trend within the industrial and commercial sphere, including in the alcohol beverage industry.

THE POLITICS OF RISK COMMUNICATION

Conflicts of Interest

Especially when it comes to the communication of risks, there is a need to ensure that any information shared is accurate and balanced, and that it is not used to misguide or promote a particular agenda. Our ability to make informed decisions hinges upon this. The integrity of scientific research and possible conflicts of interest that may compromise it are the subject of ongoing debate. Whatever the potential source of the conflict, the basic issue remains whether the information provided is accurate or whether the very results of scientific research have been skewed. The true test is still the ability of the science to speak for itself.

Conflicts of interest in research and in the area of risk analysis and communication come in many guises. Ties to corporate or industry interests are often perceived as a possible source of conflict, particularly where financial relationships are involved, including corporate sponsorship of research, corporate gifts, or a financial stake in the research by the scientists themselves. Especially in recent years, the increased overlap between the academic and private sectors through technology transfer intended to promote progress in scientific inquiry has raised concern that conflicts, financial or otherwise, may compromise the integrity of science itself (Hasselmo, 2002; Kassirer, 2001).

Research in biomedicine and technology has been clouded by concern that vested interests in the results may, at times, drive the outcomes. Experience derived from the case of the tobacco industry, in particular, has raised concerns that commercial reasons may underlie the suppression or distortion of research results (Bekelman, Li, & Gross, 2003). More recent cases involving pharmaceutical industry-funded research into the efficacy and safety of new drugs have received similar attention. Private sector funding of research, as well as consultancy arrangements between scientists and corporations, may mean that researchers themselves have a direct financial stake in the work they are conducting. The incentive to suppress negative findings, especially those that might jeopardize financial performance or patent rights, is therefore arguably strong.

Yet, other equally insidious and potentially damaging sources of conflict may affect information about risk and set the agenda for how it is communicated. These sources may have nothing to do with commercial interests or financial ties. The association with certain ideological or religious positions can drive research agendas as strongly as relationships with corporations. Whereas commercial interests are focused on selling products and swaying consumer choices, ideological interests are focused on selling a particular view of the world and on swaying public opinion. An interesting question to consider is why research linked to foundations with ties to the temperance movement, for example, should be regarded as less a source of conflict in alcohol research than relationships with a producer of beverage alcohol.

Finally, other, less tangible sources of potential conflict exist. Fierce competition in the research field and the desire for prestige or tenure among researchers may, at times, present a serious threat to the very integrity of science. Even trusted and expert sources do not come free of their own values and judgments. It is worth keeping in mind that expertise and credibility do not necessarily imply personal and moral integrity. Experts, like anyone else, can be expected to bring their own judgments to bear on the conclusions they draw.

In an effort to ensure the integrity of scientific research, several measures have been put in place over the years to disclose potential sources of conflicting interests. Most scientific and medical journals have implemented editorial policies around such disclosure, although these policies generally seek mainly disclosure of financial ties and relationships with the private sector.

The medical journal *The Lancet,* for example, has the following to say:

> Conflict of interest for a given manuscript exists when a participant in the peer review and publication process—author, reviewer, and editor—has ties to activities that could inappropriately influence his or her judgment, whether

or not judgment is in fact affected. Financial relationships with industry (for example, through employment, consultancies, stock ownership, honoraria, expert testimony), either directly or through immediate family, are usually considered to be the most important conflicts of interest. However, conflicts can occur for other reasons, such as personal relationships, academic competition, and intellectual passion.

Public trust in the peer review process and the credibility of published articles depend in part on how well conflict of interest is handled during writing, peer review, and editorial decision making. Bias can often be identified and eliminated by careful attention to the scientific methods and conclusions of the work. Financial relationships and their effects are less easily detected than other conflicts of interest. Participants in peer review and publication should disclose their conflicting interests, and the information should be made available so that others can judge their effects for themselves. Because readers may be less able to detect bias in review articles and editorials than in reports of original research, some journals do not accept reviews and editorials from authors with a conflict of interest (*The Lancet*, 2001).

Similarly, the *Journal of the American Medical Association* (2003) states in its conflict of interest policy that "[a]uthors should indicate relevant conflicts of interest, including specific financial interests relevant to the subject of their manuscript. . . . Authors without relevant financial interests in the manuscript should indicate no such interest."

Within the substance abuse field, financial relationships with the manufacturers of tobacco, alcohol, and pharmaceuticals are seen as some of the most troubling ties. The Farmington Consensus (1997), for example, drafted by collaborating editors of leading journals in the field, requires the disclosure of such ties by submitting authors. Such disclosure practices have been criticized as prejudicial to the very findings that are reported in the journals and decried as a form of censorship that prevents research being judged on its own merits (Rothman, 1993; Martinic, 2001). The concern is that the integrity of the work is condemned a priori, without being given due consideration.

An extreme example of the prejudicial nature of potential conflicts of interests is an editorial decision made in 2001 by the journal *Addiction* to revoke an article published in 1991 on the social costs of smoking (Ellemann-Jensen, 1991). At the time of its submission, the article underwent a conventional peer review process and was recommended for publication by the referees. Ten years later, the editor of *Addiction* had the following to say:

> Recently, it has come to my notice that the paper may have an undeclared tobacco industry connection. It was submitted to *Addiction* at the direct instigation of the tobacco industry.

In these circumstances, it is necessary for protection of the integrity of the
science base to state that Dr. Ellemann-Jensen's paper is herewith formally
deemed by this journal to be withdrawn from publication. It should in the
future not be cited or quoted (Edwards, 2001).

What makes this case unusual is that the actual work and results presented
by the author are not questioned. In fact, according to others who responded
to *Addiction*'s editorial decision, no exception can be taken with the findings
or the quality of the research involved (Møller Pedersen & Christiansen,
2002). Dr. Ellemann-Jensen's work was discredited based solely on the
possibility of a conflict of interest. Adding to the bizarre nature of this story
is that when the paper was published in 1991, such conflict disclosures were
not required and that Dr. Ellemann-Jensen's death during the intervening
years prevented him from defending the integrity of his work.

In a field heavily dominated by ideology and deeply held convictions
about psychoactive substances in general and the role of alcohol in society in
particular, it seems odd that editorial policies fail to address other agendas
that should be held on an equal footing with commercial ties. It can be
argued that authors in the employ of or funded by organizations with strong
ideological or religious ties also should be required to disclose these as
potential conflicts of interest. There is no reason to believe that a close relationship with the International Order of Good Templars (IOGT), Eurocare,
the Global Alcohol Policy Alliance (GAPA), Alcohol Concern, or any number of other organizations closely affiliated with the temperance movement
could not influence research findings or how information is reported.

Initial steps have been made to address this issue, but they fall short of
being sufficient. For example, the *British Medical Journal* (2003) not only
requires declarations around "competing financial interests," but also those
relating to "a deep personal or religious conviction that may have affected what
[the author] wrote and that readers should be aware of when reading [the]
paper." *The Dublin Principles of Cooperation,* a consensus document prepared
by the International Center for Alcohol Policies (ICAP) and The National
College of Ireland (1997), reflects input from scientists, industry executives,
government officials, public health experts, and individuals from intergovernmental and nongovernmental organizations in an attempt to draw guidelines
around relationships that might compromise the integrity of alcohol research.

One point, however, cannot be sufficiently stressed. It is important
to differentiate between *actual* and *potential* conflicts. Scientific findings,
including, and perhaps especially, those relating to risk information, should
be judged primarily on their intrinsic merits. The potential for conflicting
interests does not necessarily mean that anything improper has actually occurred or that the findings are in any way flawed. Ideally, in scientific research
it is ultimately the function of the peer review process to ensure that the
integrity of scientific data is safeguarded.

Moral Entrepreneurs and Public Health

Information about science and other subjects, particularly in the area of risk, is subject not only to the forces and potential conflicts already discussed, but may also be driven by another powerful agenda. Some people believe that the public at large is incapable of making its own decisions (or, at least, the *right* decisions) and that, as a result, these decisions must be made on its behalf. This category includes the so-called "moral entrepreneurs" who wage a self-appointed campaign to steer the world toward a particular ideological goal. These moral crusaders and ideologues generally view the world as a dichotomy between good and evil, kept in balance only through the creation and enforcement of rules (Becker, 1963). This type of crusade has strong social overtones. Usually, those in a stronger social or economic position are intent on helping those whom they perceive to be less fortunate, capable, or in need of guidance. Moral entrepreneurs are in the business of establishing rules based on morality; they define beliefs that run counter to theirs as deviant. Their view of the world is typically self-righteous, based on the conviction that they are actually improving others' lot in life. The motives of moral entrepreneurs are often humanitarian, driven by the strong conviction that those around them are incapable of helping themselves.

The alcohol field, with its often bitterly divided views, provides fertile ground for moral entrepreneurship. Perhaps one of the most striking historical examples is the Temperance Movement of the 19th and early 20th centuries that ultimately resulted in Prohibition in the U.S., which lasted from 1920 to 1933 (Gusfield, 1963).

The Temperance Movement, particularly as embodied in the activities of the Women's Christian Temperance Union (WCTU), represented an effort of the "old" middle class to regain the footing it had lost to a rising middle class made up of the newly rich and the immigrants who had flocked to the United States. By identifying itself with temperance, the WCTU movement found a symbol of its moral indignation in the changing order of things. This alliance defined and distinguished the lifestyle of the "old" middle class as it struggled to retain its values. This element of moral entrepreneurship, characterized by a "high-moral-ground" stance, is clearly defined in the following statement: "Status issues function as vehicles through which a non-economic group has deference conferred upon it or degradation conferred upon it. Victory in issues of status is the symbolic conferral of respect upon the norms of the victor and disrespect upon the norms of the vanquished" (Newburn, 1992, p. 44).

The legacy of this movement continues today through organizations such as the IOGT and its affiliated bodies, including Eurocare, Alcohol Concern, GAPA, and the Marin Institute for the Prevention of Alcohol and Other Drug Problems in the United States. These organizations are driven by ideology, leaving little middle ground or room for negotiation. To them, the alcohol field is a battleground, and it is their self-appointed duty to defend those whom they perceive to be in need of protection—whether their charges like it or not.

Some people hold the view that within the field of public health, in general, moral entrepreneurship has gained momentum during recent years, eroding the boundaries between medicine and politics. At a time when the world's population, on balance, is experiencing better health than ever before, people also have a greater awareness of health risks. Primarily in developed countries, this has created the concept of the "worried well"—persons who are concerned with health risks that they are not likely to experience first hand (Fitzpatrick, 2001).

For those who believe that many campaigns to communicate health risks to the public are, in effect, an example of moral entrepreneurship, these attempts at "reform" also represent a concerted effort to intrude into the private lives of individuals. Health policy is considered a tool for social control (Fitzpatrick, 2001), a means to establish norms of acceptable behavior under the guise of campaigns depicting everyone as being at risk.

Just how acceptable moral entrepreneurship may be depends on individual judgment and values; however, it does offer insight into what is required to establish trust and an identity as an expert source. Like actors on a stage, experts must present themselves to their audiences in a convincing way that will gain them acceptance as competent and credible; the ultimate goal is to persuade their audiences to reach a particular (and desired) conclusion (Hilgartner, 2000). The key to convincing one's audience appears to lie in persuasive rhetoric. Often, it is the way in which issues are framed, instead of their substance that determines their impact: "(T)hose who frame the questions often control the answers" (Shrader-Frechette, 1995). Framing is used widely in a variety of fields to magnify certain risks and to trivialize others, according to need. Framed the right way, an issue can galvanize audiences or create apathy, or downplay risks or enhance our perception of them. Rhetoric is crafted precisely for the purpose of politicizing the debate and manipulating public opinion.

In any field in which beliefs, value systems, and agendas—moral, ideological, political, or commercial—are at odds with one another, language is carefully chosen to frame issues and to either condone or condemn. The language of the alcohol policy debate is no exception. Following the repeal of Prohibition in the U.S., medical science began for a period to downplay the harmful effects of reckless alcohol consumption in authoritative scientific publications (Katcher, 1993). This trend has been attributed to a move by post-repeal scientists to distance themselves from the temperance ideology that had prevailed in the U.S. during Prohibition.

When one examines the rhetoric of the alcohol debate, it becomes clear that both "sides" of the issue use language as an inflammatory and political tool to shape perceptions and convey the risks associated with alcohol. Describing those who are employed by the alcohol industry as "booze merchants" and "legal drug pushers" paints an unsavory picture, casting them in the worst possible light (Center for Substance Abuse Prevention/ International Center for Alcohol Policies, 1998). Equally offensive is classifying as "Neoprohibitionists" those who wish to see the availability of alcohol curtailed in an effort to reduce its abuse.

COMMUNICATING RISKS—WHO TALKS AND WHO LISTENS?

> "You've got to remember that these are just simple farmers. These are people of the land. The common clay of the New West. You know—morons."
>
> *The Waco Kid,* Blazing Saddles *(1974)*

Although we may trust some sources of risk information more than others, in reality, a wide array of players is involved. As discussed, some of these players are "experts"; others are not. It is worth examining our main sources of information. After all, whether we realize it or not, they are instrumental in shaping how we perceive risks and how much (or how little) we know about the nature of these risks.

The Public Sector

When it comes to addressing risks, both real and perceived, public officials play a crucial role. These officials are part of local and national governments, responsible for ensuring the safety of the population. They include all those in the employ of government institutions with a direct role in managing risks, as well as those connected with intergovernmental organizations whose function extends beyond a single country or region.

It is the primary responsibility of these officials to provide balanced and accurate information, educating the public about potential risks and enabling them to make informed choices. It is also their role to help protect populations from health risks, and, where appropriate and necessary, to play a role in intervention, taking on the task of damage control and ensuring that the well-being of the population, if compromised, can be restored.

The communication of risk to the public is a primary responsibility of the governmental sector. The degree of government involvement and the appropriate extent of its intervention in the lives of individuals are the subject of considerable debate. The rather disparate views on this issue and their implications for policy are addressed in greater depth in Chapter 6.

In communicating risk information to the public, health officials rely on a number of criteria. They assess whether enough plausible evidence is available to make a claim that risk is present. This claim is based on an evaluation of how thoroughly evidence has been collected and documented and whether there is well-founded cause for concern. In the process, any lingering uncertainties should be acknowledged. After assessing the evidence and determining if there exists a cause for concern, public health officials need to weigh how best to respond, and, as they do so, making it clear to the public the way in which the final decision was made.

As a provider of health and risk information, government has several roles to play (Ippolito, 1999). It should encourage comprehensive and unbiased research that can contribute to our understanding of potential risks. To this end, a mechanism exists in most countries for ensuring that public funds are channeled to basic research through government institutions that make them available through a process based on fairness and the intrinsic merits of the research in question.

Another role for government involves providing expert assessments of scientific information. This function clearly hinges upon the assumption that such judgments will be made in an objective and unbiased way; however, this may not always be a valid assumption. For example, where regulation or legislation depends upon such evaluations, interested parties may have a strong incentive to influence their outcomes to suit particular agendas, not so much by interfering with the results as by influencing the composition of expert committees acting on behalf of governments (Ippolito, 1999). Where the assessment of risk is concerned, such influence may have serious consequences.

Government also plays a role in providing available and balanced knowledge to the public, which may help to shape behavior. One such example is providing nutritional information, which is available from a number of governments around the world. Such information may also include guidelines on the consumption of alcohol. Governments may also choose other modes for communicating risk information (e.g., putting warning labels on pharmaceuticals or tobacco products, alcohol content information on alcohol-containing beverages, or nutritional information on food packaging). Such preventive measures simultaneously remind consumers of potential risks and offer information to help modify their behaviors.

This approach has been applied to beverage alcohol in an effort to minimize risk and to effect a behavioral change where necessary. Official drinking guidelines often include recommendations about "safe" or "low-risk" drinking levels and risks inherent in heavy drinking, along with advice for populations deemed particularly at risk or, in some cases, for whom drinking may carry particular benefits. Guidelines can also include information about other activities that, when combined with alcohol consumption, may result in increased risk for harm, such as driving or operating heavy machinery (International Center for Alcohol Policies [ICAP], 2003a).

As with all risk information, the crafting of drinking guidelines relies on a thorough assessment of the best available scientific evidence. Even so, little consensus exists across guidelines regarding "safe" levels of drinking.

For instance, the official Canadian guidelines place the recommended daily levels of consumption at 27.2 grams of pure ethanol for both men and women, while the Slovenian government's recommended levels are up to 50 grams for men and 30 grams for women, and the New Zealand government suggests 60 grams and 40 grams for men and women, respectively (ICAP, 2003b). The regional government of the Basque Country in Spain, on the other hand, raises the bar even higher, with guidelines of up to 70 grams daily for men and women. To complicate matters even further, no standard exists for a "standard" drink, where the size and alcohol content cover a broad range (Martinic, 2000).

One specific focus of many official government-issued guidelines on alcohol consumption is on "special" populations who, for a number of reasons, are advised either not to drink or to do so with caution (ICAP, 2001b). These generally include children and young people, and those with a particular genetic or medical vulnerability to the effects of alcohol, such as pregnant women or the elderly. Because of differences in their physiology and alcohol metabolism, women are generally advised to consume alcohol at lower levels than men.

Having weighed the same body of evidence, governments may arrive at different conclusions about how risk information should be interpreted. The majority of countries that issue cautionary recommendations for alcohol advise against drinking during pregnancy (ICAP, 1999). A few countries, however, advise against intoxication and recommend not complete abstinence but a lower level of consumption (Royal College of Obstetricians and Gynaecologists, 1999).

So, why the differences? Several reasons factor into the evaluation and interpretation of risk information regarding alcohol. The first is culture, a potent influence in how different governments view risks and provide information about them. The role of culture in risk perception, particularly as it relates to alcohol, was discussed in depth in Chapter 2. It is evident that alcohol plays a unique role in different societies; it is acceptable in some and less acceptable in others. These attitudes are certainly reflected in government recommendations, as well as in how scientific evidence is interpreted and applied.

Another factor to consider is the nature of government-issued messages. By necessity, official recommendations are aimed at entire populations, leaving little room for individual differences. As a result, such recommendations must be general enough to apply to everyone within a given population, making the target usually the "lowest common denominator." Because recommendations are designed to apply to all possible eventualities, there is also a tendency to err on the side of caution.

Governments have been criticized for simplifying messages and for not trusting individuals to make the right decisions for themselves. Yet, it can be argued that it is not the place of government to tailor risk information to individual needs. Instead, it is up to individuals and to those who provide them with information and counsel (e.g., their physicians) to extrapolate from official recommendations and to apply risk information in a way that is appropriate to the particular instance and lifestyle at hand.

Numerous other factors play a role in the way governments provide risk information to the public, specifically in the areas of nutrition and health. Any recommendations made in dietary (or drinking) guidelines have implications for health programs, future research, and, last but not least, consumer choices. How recommendations are worded can have considerable impact on all these areas; thus, wording is also carefully monitored by the industries potentially affected by both positive and negative recommendations (Nestle, 1996). Because of their highly influential role in providing risk information, governments need to maintain a fine balance when communicating news of both risks and benefits.

Health Professionals

A one-size-fits-all message about health concerns and risk information cannot adequately provide specific guidance to individuals who differ from one another in health status and lifestyle. Information on potential risks must be balanced against potential benefits for each individual. What is required, therefore, is the ability to distill available information on risk and to apply it to individual cases.

Providing balanced information on risks potentially associated with alcohol consumption presents a challenge to health professionals. Although heavy and otherwise problematic drinking can carry serious health, social, and psychological consequences, research has also shown that moderate alcohol consumption may carry with it health benefits not only for coronary heart disease, but also for other areas of health (Grant & Litvak, 1998; MacDonald, 1999). Before any recommendation is given, the individual circumstances must be weighed carefully because there is an obligation to provide patients with a full and accurate picture of both the benefits and risks involved (Klatsky, 1999).

Such recommendations to individuals are best provided by physicians, to whom we turn for advice on matters of health. For many people, the family practitioner represents the primary point of contact with the health care professional, and thus represents an ideal point of intervention and a useful vehicle for providing risk information. The argument for this pivotal role is strengthened by the view held by most people that the family physician is an appropriate and trusted source for advice. Others, however, often serve as the primary point of health care contact for many people around the world: nurses and other trained staff who provide medical care and health information, or pharmacists whose advice is often sought by the public. Their role in health care is a critical one; it is also potentially crucial in providing risk information.

In practice, evidence exists that physicians may not adequately provide advice on alcohol consumption. A recent study found that 94% of physicians fail to detect the symptoms of alcohol abuse among their patients (Graham, Maio, Blow, & Hill, 2000). Two main reasons support this criticism:

1. Many physicians lack the necessary skills and training to discuss risky drinking and potential harm with their patients (Miller, Sheppard, Colenda, & Magen, 2001).
2. Physicians may be consulted or asked to intervene only after problems have already developed.

This may be attributable, in part, to higher priority given to other behaviors with a potential impact on health, such as smoking, exercise, safe sex, or nutrition. It has also been argued that the moral implications and social values associated with substance abuse, particularly with the role of drinking in different societies, present an obstacle to the involvement of physicians (Chappel & Lewis, 1999).

A survey of clinicians conducted in New Zealand suggests that fewer than 25% of those questioned had received adequate training in diagnosing alcohol problems correctly and offering appropriate intervention (Alcohol Advisory Council of New Zealand, 1999a). As a result, only a small fraction of patients with alcohol problems are diagnosed and offered intervention and treatment (Klamen, 1999). Similar inadequacies in physician training also exist in other countries, leading not only to failure to diagnose, but also to problems that may be misdiagnosed or even overdiagnosed, as well as advice on drinking that is not accurately presented (Owens, Gilmore, & Pirmohamed, 2000)

The case of fetal alcohol syndrome (FAS) provides a good example. FAS is a condition occurring in the children of women whose alcohol consumption during pregnancy is heavy and chronic. These children exhibit a number of distinctive physical characteristics, as well as brain damage (Streissguth & O'Malley, 2000; Warren et al., 2001). In most industrialized countries, FAS occurs at a rate of 1 or 2 in every 1,000 live births. The highest incidence of FAS in any nation in the world has been reported in the U.S., a rate 20 times higher than that in the rest of the world combined (Abel, 1995). In countries such as France, Spain, and Italy, where alcohol consumption levels are higher than in the U.S., however, cases of FAS are virtually nonexistent (Abel, 1998).

It has been speculated that part of the reason for this disparity may be the eagerness with which U.S. physicians diagnose FAS (Abel, 1995). Because the condition is extremely rare, medical training may not be adequate to allow accurate diagnosis, instead relying primarily on the identification of facial features. In an ethnically heterogeneous society, Abel claims, ethnic characteristics may be misinterpreted as features of FAS.

There may be another dimension to the rate at which FAS is diagnosed. Heightened sensitivity to the issue exists in the U.S., where FAS is regarded as a social problem (Armstrong & Abel, 2000). The prominence given to FAS may well be a reflection of the general perception of risks associated with alcohol in U.S. culture.

A further argument for this interpretation is an analysis conducted on the incidence of spontaneous abortions attributed to very low levels of drinking during pregnancy (Abel, 1997). Virtually every study supporting such a relationship has been carried out in the U.S. or Canada, while those in which such a link has not been corroborated have been conducted in Australia or Europe. This discrepancy argues in favor of a cultural impact on risk assessment and its reflection on medical training and diagnosis. Recent trends in medical education suggest that such views may be changing and that information about alcohol, both the risks and health benefits, is being added to medical school curricula (Chappel & Lewis, 1999) and directed at various medical specialties.

Efforts have also been made to educate other health providers about alcohol. In many countries in which health care is inaccessible or unaffordable to the majority of the population, the pharmacist functions as a primary point of contact with the health profession and can play a key role in providing risk information relating to lifestyle, including alcohol consumption. This relationship has proved to be a useful approach to delivering information about alcohol. In Chile, for example, pharmacists across the country have been trained to recognize symptoms of alcohol abuse among their clients. They share health and risk information with the customers they serve, and provide behavioral and lifestyle counseling in an attempt to modify behavior (Zunino, Litvak, & Israel, 1998).

Health professionals involved in risk communication also include a range of other players who generate information and offer advice for the public at large. These include professional societies and associations, such as those representing the medical profession and its various subdisciplines. They also include various nongovernmental organizations involved in communicating health and risk information: "consumer watchdog groups" and advocacy groups concerned with health issues. The latter organizations are frequently permeated by moral entrepreneurship, and their agendas are reflected in the information they provide.

THE PRIVATE SECTOR AND RISK COMMUNICATION

Over the years, awareness that risk is an important issue for the public has been growing within the private sector. Good corporate citizenship includes not only the responsible marketing of products, but also the reduction of potential harms that might be associated with them. The private sector is quick to learn from the mistakes of the past. The path taken by the tobacco industry and its apparent efforts to hide risk information about its products have been recognized as mistakes to be avoided at all costs.

In order to be viable, private enterprise needs to focus on maximizing profits. As a result, its approaches to risk communication may, at times, differ from those employed by the public sector, which is not profit-driven. Although both sources may take on the function of informing the public, the private sector may also wish to use risk communication to influence outcomes (Taig, 1999). For example, by stressing their safety records, industries can sway public opinions and, ultimately, consumer choices. Risk information can be used to differentiate a company from its competitors by pointing to differences in risk management. Demand by the public for full and balanced risk information has also resulted in an increased industry commitment to risk research and to addressing the public's concerns.

Similar to other industries marketing products that, when misused, have a potential for harm, the beverage alcohol industry has made an effort to address the concerns of consumers regarding risks. Much of this information is imparted through education about responsible drinking and ways to reduce harm from irresponsible and problematic alcohol consumption. In a number of countries, special industry-funded bodies have been set up with the sole purpose of providing risk information and educating consumers about responsible drinking and risky behavior. These bodies, known as social aspects organizations (SAOs), are active in several countries in Europe and North America, as well as in Africa and Asia.

The activities of most SAOs are focused primarily in areas in which risk information is particularly helpful, including drunk driving and the education of populations that are particularly vulnerable (e.g., young people). SAO efforts to promote information about potential risks associated with particular drinking patterns include campaigns that are likely to engage the attention and interest of their audiences. For example, The Portman Group in the United Kingdom and The Century Council in the U.S. provide calculator-like devices and computer programs designed to inform young people about levels and patterns of drinking and the risks associated with reckless and heavy alcohol consumption (The Century Council, 2003; The Portman Group, 2003).

Other SAOs, including the German organization known as DIFA Forum, provide information about drinking in the workplace and drinking during pregnancy (DIFA Forum, 2003). SAOs, such as the Danish GODA, the Dutch STIVA, and the Polish MODUS, have developed informational materials for use in the classroom in an effort to apply the lifeskills approach to educating young people about risks associated with drinking. An overview of SAO activities in Europe is offered on the website of The Amsterdam Group (The Amsterdam Group, 2003). In South Africa, whose Western Cape region has the highest single localized incidence of fetal alcohol syndrome in the world (Crawford & Viljoen, 1999; Viljoen, 1999; May et al., 2000), the

SAO ARA (Association for Responsible Alcohol Consumption, 2003) has undertaken efforts to promote research on this issue and to educate the local population about risks and behaviors. Where the availability of noncommercially produced alcohol is widespread, efforts have also been made to provide information about the risk of poisoning by methanol and other toxic additives.

Although many alcohol industry initiatives are implemented through SAOs and other bodies, including national trade associations, many individual companies also have programs and campaigns designed to educate consumers about responsible drinking. In addition, most companies provide guidelines and information specifically aimed at their employees, many of whom are in constant contact with alcohol in the workplace and require full and balanced information about potential risks (ICAP, 2003a). Moreover, the codes of practice to which the marketing of beverage alcohol is held in many parts of the world are implemented to ensure that the representation of alcohol by industry is accurate and does not mislead the consumer about potential risks. Many of these codes are attempts by the industry to regulate itself and to minimize potential risks associated with its products (ICAP, 2001a).

THE ROLE OF THE MEDIA

No discussion of risk communication is complete without addressing the role of the media. In today's world, many people rely on media outlets, particularly radio and television, to provide information on issues affecting their lives. Given the habits of different societies, it is likely that these figures and their implications for the dissemination of information vary significantly. In developing countries, television, where available, and radio are sources of information about virtually any topic from current events to health information. For those living in the relative affluence of developed countries, particularly for younger individuals, the Internet has joined the more traditional media as a key source of information.

The results of a study carried out for the Health Protection and Consumer Protection Directorate-General (DG-SANCO) of the European Commission shows that nearly one in four Europeans (23%) use the Internet as a source of health information (Spadaro, 2003). Differences exist across countries. In Denmark and the Netherlands, about 40% of people use the Internet to access information, while in Greece, Spain, Portugal, and France, only 15% or fewer turn to the Internet as a resource. However, the study also found that for most Europeans, doctors and pharmacists constitute the main source of health information, and that the traditional media are still used with greater frequency than the Internet. The results of another study suggest that although men are more likely to use the Internet for general information, women are more likely to turn to it for information on health (Datamonitor, 2002).

Although the media may be a potent tool for communicating risk information and raising awareness of hazards, the fundamental question is: What role *should* the media play? Is it the responsibility of the media to educate the public? If so, what and how much information should the media provide? Or, is the media's role simply one of delivering the kind of information the public wants?

The role of the media has been discussed at length. With regard to the media's role in reporting about alcohol issues, four main functions have been suggested: advertising, education, stories that relate alcohol and drinking to everyday life, and provision of a forum in which issues relevant to alcohol policy can be discussed (Partanen, 1988). These portrayals of alcohol as it fits in with daily life are closely related to the socializing role of the mass media. Another question is whether media portrayals are a reflection of attitudes and culture or whether they are instrumental in shaping attitudes and culture (Anglin, Johnson, Giesbrecht, & Greenfield, 2000; Lemmens, Vaeth, & Greenfield, 1999). Some have argued that media portrayals of alcohol issues, particularly when it comes to risk, reflect the views of journalists themselves, a group with a generally heavier pattern of drinking than found in other professions (Baillie, 1996; Plant, 1986).

It can be argued, however, that the media are responsible only for reporting, and that it is incumbent upon us, the consumers of media information, to keep these caveats in mind. It is up to the public to draw its own conclusions, just as it is up to others to enlighten. Whatever the media's role, they are powerful providers of risk information, be it accurate and balanced or steeped in bias, myth, or misinformation.

Writing about the media in the 1920s, columnist Walter Lippmann noted that because most of what people "know" about the world around them comes not from personal experience but from mass media, there is a danger of confusing reality with the *reporting* of reality, a creation by intermediaries (in this case, journalists) (Lippmann, 1922). Lippmann's note of caution is well taken. The media represent an additional layer of translation between the source of the news and the audience, often coloring the way in which information is presented. It is important to bear in mind, especially when addressing risk information, that journalists are generally not scientists. They may lack the skills to fully understand what they are reporting, may need to cut corners in order to meet a deadline, or may rely on a small number of experts whose input is repeatedly sought, thus creating an oligarchy of "trusted sources" that may not always be the most credible. It is important to keep these caveats in mind to avoid a dangerous blurring of lines and not to lose sight of the fact that the media are but a filter. The following example illustrates this point.

In 1998, a study carried out at the Harvard School of Public Health examined the relationship between alcohol consumption in women and the incidence of breast cancer (Smith-Warner et al., 1998). The study was particularly noteworthy because it analyzed data from more than 300,000 women pooled from a number of earlier independent studies. The conclusions of this meta-analysis suggested that although alcohol consumption could raise the risk of breast cancer in women over a lifetime, this increase in risk was very small. In women who drank at low to moderate levels, the increase was especially small and, at some levels, even lower than for abstainers. In heavier drinkers, on the other hand, the risk for breast cancer was increased over that for nondrinkers.

The newsworthiness of these findings and their general interest to the public were picked up by the media, and many newspapers ran the story. However, as the media filtered the basic information and reduced it to something easily accessible to the general readership, the message became oversimplified—that alcohol consumption increases the risk of breast cancer. The typical resulting news story focused on this single piece of information. The reporting of the findings was generally not accompanied by necessary caveats, namely that increases in risk were associated only with heavier drinking, not with moderate alcohol consumption in women, and that other factors, such as a family history of breast cancer, were strong determinants of outcomes for the individual.

Of the 12 stories (see the following headlines) reporting on the findings of the study on February 18, 1998, only 2 acknowledged that the increased risk in question was related primarily to heavy alcohol consumption:

> "Alcohol linked to breast cancer"; "Alcohol, cancer linked"; "Heavy drinking is reported to boost breast cancer risk"; "Alcohol increases risk of breast cancer"; "Alcohol is linked to breast cancer"; "Study links alcohol, risk of breast cancer"; "More than 2 drinks a day said to boost risk"; "Study links daily alcohol, breast cancer"; " Studies confirm relationship of alcohol to breast cancer"; "Alcohol tie to breast cancer affirmed"; "Study links alcohol to breast cancer risk"; "Daily drink may up breast cancer risk."[1]

Part of the difficulty in translating complex results of scientific research is that the media tend to deal with implied numbers and values. Risks are often conveyed in qualitative terms such as "very high," "negligible," and "safe." Little, if any, accompanying information is available regarding what these values signify. Just how negligible is "negligible?" What does it mean for the behavior and lifestyle of those reading the report? Chapter 3 addresses the issue of risk assessment and the interpretation of risk information in detail.

---

[1]These February 18, 1998, headlines, in order of appearance, were taken from the following sources: *The Toronto Star*, News, p. A20; *Sacramento Bee*, Main News, p. A8; *The [Cleveland] Plain Dealer*, National, p. 10A; *The Ottawa Citizen*, News, p. A13; *The Daily Telegraph*, p. 5; *The Buffalo News*, News, p. 4A; *The Boston Herald*, News, p. 5; *Chicago Tribune*, News, p. 11; *The New York Times*, Section A, p. 16; *The Boston Globe*, National/Foreign, p. A3; *The Arizona Republic*, Front, p. A8; *Chicago Sun-Times*, Food, p. 2.

Earlier, this chapter discussed conflicts of interest and the potential impact of hidden agendas on the communication of risk. Similar to other sectors, the media are not immune to such forces. Media outlets may have particular biases, which can be government-imposed, economically motivated, or driven by a special ideology. The following pointers on how information, particularly medical and risk information, should be conveyed to and interpreted by the public offer helpful guidance:

1. An association between two events is not the same as cause and effect.
2. Demonstrating one link in a chain of events does not prove the whole chain.
3. Probabilities are not the same as certainties.
4. The framing of scientific results can affect their impact (Angell & Kassirer, 1994).

Audiences

Audiences for risk information span many different groups, each with its own set of requirements and ability to receive and use the information presented. The following hierarchy of audiences has been suggested, some more closely involved than others in the process of risk communication (Miller, 1987):

- At the top of the hierarchy are the decision makers. Typically, they represent government (local, national, and global) and are involved in making and controlling policy decisions. Although this group may be a provider of risk information to the public, it is also an audience receiving information from its original sources, such as the scientists who determine and analyze risks.

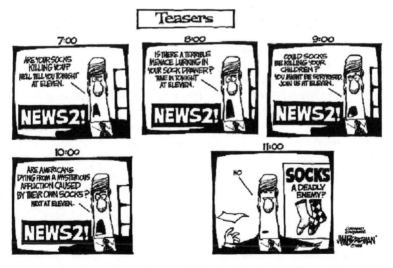

Copyright 5/20/98 Jim Borgman, *Cincinnati Enquirer.* Reprinted with special permission of King Features Syndicate.

- The next group consists of nongovernment policy leaders, who do not actually make decisions but provide advice during the decision-making process and also have the ear of the public.
- The bulk of the audience consists of the public, which can be divided into two basic groups. The first is the "attentive" public, those who are attuned to the policy-making process and are able to influence decision makers by direct contact and political persuasion. They include the political activists who are involved in the process, but without official status. The second, and larger, group consists of the "non-attentive" public—those with a limited understanding of science and policy and the formulation of risk decisions. It is important to note that "non-attentive" does not mean ignorant. Instead, individuals in this group (likely 70–80% of the general population) may be interested in certain areas and issues and uninterested in others.

Studies have claimed that the public at large is incapable of grasping complicated concepts and understanding nuances and that it cannot be trusted to make its own judgments. The reality is that the public is generally reluctant to follow advice on risks unless this advice is directly relevant to them as individuals. This does not mean, however, that the public does not comprehend the information presented to it. Although the public at large may not be well versed in the intricacies of science or sufficiently sophisticated to interpret complex probabilities and mathematical relationships, the notion that most people are uninterested in what goes on in the world around them is simply not true. "Ordinary" people have an inherent interest in science; it touches their everyday lives. Science is not an arcane discipline, impenetrable to the uninitiated, or some sort of secret society from which the public at large is barred.

Hard-to-Reach Populations

Even in this age of technological advances and globalization, much of the world's population continues to live in poverty. "If we get a road we would get everything else: community center, employment, post office, water, telephone" (The World Bank, 2000). This quote from Jamaica illustrates how access to necessities also opens the door to greater access to information. For those faced with a need for fundamental resources in life, adequate communication of risk remains a challenging proposition.

Mainstream approaches may be largely ineffective in disseminating risk information to many hard-to-reach populations. In such instances, creative and novel channels need to be found and relied on because it is those who have the least access to conventional means that may be vulnerable to the greatest risks, be they health epidemics or natural disasters. In addition, as discussed in Chapter 2, cultural differences often create barriers to the effective communication of risk information.

Innovative techniques have been developed to spread the word about public health risks and stem the spread of infection. Particularly in the area of HIV/AIDS, new approaches are helping to slow the spread of infection. One such approach, implemented in a number of countries, including India, is the education of remote rural populations about the risk of HIV transmission. A professional troupe of actors travels from village to village, offering health information in the form of a dramatic presentation, educating and entertaining at the same time. When dramatized in this way, topics that may otherwise represent cultural taboos can suddenly be discussed. The approach also allows information to be shared with those who are illiterate or do not have access to other communication channels or to health care providers (Koninklijk Instituut voor de Troopen, 2003; Nalamdana, 2003).

Similar approaches to raising AIDS awareness have been implemented elsewhere. In Cambodia, AIDS workers confronted with the challenges of poverty, low awareness about AIDS and condoms, and a poor infrastructure have resorted to puppet shows, one of the oldest traditional art forms in Cambodian culture, to disseminate information. Puppet shows travel around the country dramatizing their cautionary tale while, at the same time, informing audiences and debunking myths. Similar to theater troupes in India and elsewhere, Cambodian puppets, through the roles they play, have more freedom to be outspoken about topics that are generally considered taboo (Laurentin, 2002).

Where radio and television may be accessible but levels of literacy are low, other approaches have been used. A popular weekly soap opera broadcast by television stations brings messages about the spread of AIDS to the population of Côte d'Ivoire (Population Services International, 2003). Mobile video vans travel the countryside of Bangladesh delivering instructional messages on AIDS, family planning, and child care (United Nations Educational, Scientific and Cultural Organization, 2003). These alternative approaches to risk communication make use of creative techniques to educate people who might otherwise not have access to risk information.

Although these examples illustrate creative approaches to addressing disease and epidemics, they can be equally applied to a range of potentially risky behaviors, including alcohol abuse. One such approach is a "lifeskills" program implemented in primary schools in South Africa and Botswana, providing children with information about alcohol consumption and abuse within the context of a number of different issues likely to face them, including sex, drugs, and violence (ICAP, 2000). These integrated programs in schools, both in remote and in urban areas, help equip children without family and other support to address issues they will ultimately confront.

SUMMARY

So, is risk communication effective? It can be. Its effectiveness hinges upon several factors. Risk communication to the public should be a routine endeavor, an integral part of implementing any regulation or prevention approach. To be effective, all stakeholders should be allowed to play a part in formulating the risk message, determining the most effective communication processes, and finding the appropriate solutions. This means involving national and local governments, the private sector, and, last but not least, the public—an approach further discussed in Chapter 6 on policy. An effective message of risk is one that is comprehensible and tailored to its intended audience. It should be framed in a way that will resonate well and make an impression if it is to effect behavioral changes (Taig, 1999).

Risk communication, presented in a relevant and easily comprehended way, has been quite successful at effecting changes in certain behaviors. In the mid-1970s, the Department of Transportation in the United Kingdom adopted a communications campaign aimed at drunk drivers. Using television as its preferred medium, this campaign targeted young drivers, who are more likely to be at risk, by raising social concern about the issue and applying pressure to offenders. As a result, a significant change in attitudes was observed in the period between 1985 and 1995 (Taig, 1999). The campaign brought about an approximate 50% drop in drunk-driving fatalities, as well as a general shift in attitudes about acceptable behaviors, including the concept of "designated drivers" and the need to limit alcohol consumption when driving. This is but one example of the effectiveness of risk communication, but it illustrates the point: Communicating information about risks, if done properly, can alter our perception and change behavior.

It is important to emphasize that although the roles of the various sectors involved in risk communication have been addressed individually, they cannot work in isolation. Studies have demonstrated that a synergistic approach that uses a variety of channels for risk communication can be considerably more effective than isolated approaches, and multiple efforts to convey a message will ultimately reinforce one another. The usefulness of this multifaceted approach in crafting policy around risks is the topic of Chapter 6.

This chapter has attempted to paint as comprehensive a picture as possible on how risk information is presented to us and by whom. It has also examined other less obvious forces that can influence the information we are given. How we perceive the information presented to us, whether we accept or reject it, and how we relate it to our individual experience was discussed at length in Chapter 1. Many factors need to be taken into account when evaluating information on risks. As long as we are aware of some of the pitfalls, navigating the risks around us and making sense of what we are told becomes an easier task.

Some basic ground rules are needed for the effective communication of risks. Disseminating too much information at one time can cloud the issue. Information and definitions need to be comprehensible and relevant to the everyday experience of individuals. Furthermore, definitions used for scientific purposes should be kept separate from those used in common parlance, or, at the very least, explained. Unless the distinction between the two is clear, the result may be a misinformed and confused public. Information on risk should be balanced, reflecting best practice on all sides of the issue, acknowledging any gaps, uncertainties, and conflicting evidence. It should be based on verifiable evidence. Moreover, risk information should ideally be free from value judgments and include just the facts—no more and no less. For those providing information on risk, the golden rule should be to not mislead. Finally, the public should be provided with the necessary tools to make up its own mind and formulate educated decisions based on balanced evidence. Even the nonexperts among us are capable of understanding complex information if it is properly presented.

REFERENCES

Abel, E. L. (1995). An update on incidence of FAS: FAS is not an equal opportunity birth defect. *Neurotoxicology and Teratology, 17,* 437–443.

Abel, E. L. (1997). Maternal alcohol consumption and spontaneous abortion. *Alcohol and Alcoholism, 32,* 211–219.

Abel, E. L. (1998). Fetal alcohol syndrome: The "American paradox." *Alcohol and Alcoholism, 33,* 195–201.

Alcohol Advisory Council of New Zealand (ALAC). (1999a). Message reception and comprehension. In *Best practice guidelines worldwide for information services concerned with safe drinking.* Wellington: Author.

Alcohol Advisory Council of New Zealand. (1999b). Alcohol intervention in primary health care. In *Best practice guidelines worldwide for information services concerned with safe drinking.* Wellington: Author.

The Amsterdam Group. (2003). *The Amsterdam Group: The European forum for responsible drinking.* Retrieved August 19, 2003, from http://www.amsterdamgroup.org.

Angell, M., & Kassirer, J. (1994). Clinical research—What should the public believe? *New England Journal of Medicine, 331,* 189–190.

Anglin, L., Johnson, S., Giesbrecht, N., & Greenfield, T. (2000). Alcohol policy content analysis: A comparison of public health and alcohol industry trade newsletters. *Drug and Alcohol Review, 19,* 203–212.

Armstrong, E. M., & Abel, E. L. (2000). Fetal alcohol syndrome: The origins of a moral panic. *Alcohol and Alcoholism, 35,* 276–282.

Association for Responsible Alcohol Consumption. (2003). Retrieved October 28, 2003, from http://www.ara.co.za/Main.htm.

Baillie, R. K. (1996). Determining the effects of media portrayals of alcohol: Going beyond short term influence. *Alcohol and Alcoholism, 31,* 235–242.

Becker, H. S. (1963). *Outsiders: Studies in the sociology of deviance.* New York: Free Press.

Bekelman, J. E., Li, Y., & Gross, C. (2003). Scope and impact of financial conflicts of interest in biomedical research: A systematic review. *Journal of the American Medical Association, 289,* 454–465.

Borchelt, R. (2001). *And all the spaces in between: The changing role of institution-based science communication.* Paper presented at the annual meeting of the American Association for the Advancement of Science (AAAS), San Francisco, CA.

British Medical Journal. (2003). *BMJ declaration of competing interests.* Retrieved August 19, 2003, from http://bmj.com/cgi/content/full/317/7154/291/DC1.

Center for Substance Abuse Prevention/International Center for Alcohol Policies. (1998). *What do others hear when we speak about alcohol?* Working Papers. Washington, DC: Author.

The Century Council. (2003). *The blood alcohol educator.* Retrieved August 19, 2003, from http://www.b4udrink.org.

Chappel, J. N., & Lewis, D. C. (1999). Medical education. In M. Galanter & H. D. Kleber (Eds.), *Textbook of substance abuse treatment* (2nd ed., pp. 529–534). Washington, DC: American Psychiatric Press.

Crawford, J., & Viljoen, D. L. (1999). Alcohol consumption by pregnant women in the Western Cape. *South African Medical Journal, 89,* 962–965.

Datamonitor. (2002). *Who is looking for health information online? A segmentation analysis of the online consumer* (Brief No. BFHC0470). London: Author.

Delacôte, G. (1987). Science and scientists: Public perception and attitudes. In D. Evered & M. O'Connor (Eds.), *Communicating science to the public* (pp. 41–48). Chichester, UK: John Wiley & Sons.

DIFA Forum. (2003). Retrieved October 28, 2003, from http://www.difa-forum.de.

Edwards, G. (2001). A paper which must be withdrawn from publication (editorial note). *Addiction, 96,* 1099.

Ellemann-Jensen, P. (1991). The social costs of smoking revisited. *Addiction, 86,* 957–966.

The Farmington Consensus. (1997). *Addiction, 92*(12), 1617–1618.

Fitzpatrick, M. (2001). *The tyranny of health: Doctors and the regulation of lifestyle.* London: Routledge.

Frewer, L. J., Howard, C., Hedderley, D., & Sheperd, R. (1996). What determines trust in information about food-related risks? Underlying psychological constructs. *Risk Analysis, 16,* 473–486.

Frewer, L. J., Howard, C., Hedderley, D., & Sheperd, R. (1998). Methodological approaches to assessing risk perceptions associated with food-related hazards. *Risk Analysis, 18,* 95–102.

Graham, D. M., Maio, R. F., Blow, F. C., & Hill, E. M. (2000). Emergency physician attitudes concerning intervention for alcohol abuse/dependence delivered in the emergency department: A brief report. *Journal of Addictive Diseases, 19,* 45–53.

Grant, M., & Litvak, J. (1998). *Drinking patterns and their consequences.* Washington, DC: Taylor & Francis.

Gusfield, J. (1963). *Symbolic crusade: Status politics and the American temperance movement.* Urbana, IL: University of Illinois Press.

Hasselmo, N. (2002). Individual and institutional conflict of interest: Policy review by research universities in the United States. *Science and Engineering Ethics, 8,* 421–427.

Heath, D. B. (1995). *International handbook on alcohol and culture.* Westport, CT: Greenwood Press.

Heath, D. B. (2000). *Drinking occasions: Comparative perspectives on alcohol and culture.* Philadelphia, PA: Brunner/Mazel.

Heath, D. B. (2001). Culture and substance abuse. *Cultural Psychiatry: International Perspectives, 24,* 479–495.

Hilgartner, S. (2000). *Science on stage: Expert advice as public drama.* Stanford, CA: Stanford University Press.

International Center for Alcohol Policies (ICAP) and The National College of Ireland. (1997). *The Dublin Principles of Cooperation.* Washington, DC: Author.

ICAP. (1999). *Government policies on alcohol and pregnancy* (Report No. 6). Washington, DC: Author.

ICAP. (2000). *Lifeskills education in Botswana and South Africa.* Washington, DC: Author.

ICAP. (2001a). *Self-regulation of beverage alcohol advertising* (Report No. 9). Washington, DC: Author.

ICAP. (2001b). *Alcohol and special populations: Biological vulnerability* (Report No. 10). Washington, DC: Author.

ICAP. (2003a). *Alcohol and the workplace* (Report No. 13). Washington, DC: Author.
ICAP. (2003b). *International Drinking Guidelines* (Report No. 14). Washington, DC: Author.
Ippolito, P. M. (1999). How government policies shape the food and nutrition information environment. *Food Policy, 24,* 295–306.
Johnson, B. B., & Slovic, P. (1994). "Improving" risk communication and risk management: Legislated solutions or legislated disaster? *Risk Analysis, 14,* 905–906.
Journal of the American Medical Association (JAMA). (2003). *Instructions for authors. Conflict of interest policy.* Retrieved August 19, 2003, from http://jama.ama-assn.org/ifora_current.dtl.
Kaiser Family Foundation & Agency for Healthcare Research and Quality. (1996). *Americans as health care consumers: The role of quality information* (Publication 1203). Menlo Park, CA: Author.
Kassirer, J. P. (2001). Financial conflict of interest: An unresolved ethical frontier. *American Journal of Law and Medicine, 27,* 149–162.
Katcher, B. S. (1993). The post-repeal eclipse in knowledge about the harmful effects of alcohol. *Addiction, 88,* 729–744.
Katinic, K., Thaller, V., & Marusic, S. (2000). Alcohol and media. *Alcoholism: Journal on Alcoholism and Related Addictions, 36,* 87–92 .
Klamen, D. L. (1999). Education and training in addictive diseases. *Psychiatric Clinics of North America, 22,* 471–480.
Klatsky, A. (1999). Is drinking healthy? In S. Peele & M. Grant (Eds.), *Alcohol and pleasure: A health perspective* (pp. 141–156). Philadelphia, PA: Brunner/Mazel.
Koninklijk Instituut voor de Troopen [Royal Tropical Institute]. (July 2003). *Theatre & development—theatre groups.* Retrieved August 20, 2003, from http://www.kit.nl/specials/html/td_theatre_groups.as.
The Lancet. (2001). Uniform requirements for manuscripts submitted to biomedical journals. Retrieved August 19, 2003, from http://www.thelancet.com/info/info.isa?n1=authorinfo&n2=Uniform+requirements.
Langford, I. H., Marris, C., & O'Riordan, T. (1999). Public reactions to risk: Social structures, images of science and roles of trust. In P. Bennet & K. Calman (Eds.), *Risk communication and public health* (pp. 3–50). New York: Oxford University Press.
Laurentin, F. (2002). The puppet, the pencil and the condom: UNESCO's edutainment experiences in Phnom Penh. *Sexual Health Exchange, 1.* Retrieved August 20, 2003, from http://www.kit.nl/ils/exchange_content/html/puppets_hiv_aids_-sexual_healt.asp.
Lemmens, P. H., Vaeth, P. A. C., & Greenfield, T. K. (1999). Coverage of beverage alcohol issues in the print media in the United States. *American Journal of Public Health, 89,* 1555–1560.
Lippmann, W. (1922/1965). *Public opinion.* New York: Free Press.
MacDonald, I. (Ed.). (1999). *Health issues related to alcohol consumption* (2nd ed.). Oxford: Blackwell Science.
Martinic, M. (1999). Is "hazardous" drinking a useful concept for public health recommendations? *Contemporary Drug Problems, 26,* 653–672.
Martinic, M. (2000). What is a "standard drink?" In D. B. Cooper (Ed.), *Alcohol use.* Abingdon, UK: Radcliffe Medical Press.
Martinic, M. (2001). The research community and the private sector: A hands-on or hands-off relationship? *Alcoholism: Clinical and Experimental Research, 25,* 1801–1804.
May, P. A., Brooke, L., Gossage, J. P., Croxford, J., Adams, C., Jones, K. L., et al. (2000). Epidemiology of fetal alcohol syndrome in a South African community in the Western Cape province. *American Journal of Public Health, 90,* 1905–1912.

Miller, J. D. (1987). Scientific literacy in the United States. In D. Evered & M. O'Connor (Eds.), *Communicating science to the public* (pp. 19–40). Chichester, UK: John Wiley & Sons.

Miller, N. S., Sheppard, L. M., Colenda, C. C., & Magen, J. (2001). Why physicians are unprepared to treat patients who have alcohol and drug-related disorders. *Academic Medicine, 76,* 410–418.

Møller Pedersen, K., & Christiansen, T. (2002). A fair hearing or academic kangaroo court? *Addiction, 97,* 227–232.

Nalamdana. (2003). *Evaluating drama that imparts information.* Retrieved August 27, 2003, from http://www.nalamdana.org/drama.htm.

National Cancer Institute. (1984). *Cancer prevention awareness survey* (Report No. NIH, Publication No. 84-26-77). Washington, DC: Government Printing Office.

Nestle, M. (1996). Alcohol guidelines for chronic disease prevention: From prohibition to moderation. *Social History of Alcohol Review, 32–33,* 45–59.

Newburn, T. (1992) *Permission and regulation: Law and morals in post-war Britain.* London: Routledge.

Owens, L., Gilmore, I. T., & Pirmohamed, M. (2000). General practice nurses' knowledge of alcohol use and misuse: A questionnaire survey. *Alcohol & Alcoholism, 35,* 259–262.

Partanen, J. (1988, Summer). Communicating about alcohol in the mass media. *Contemporary Drug Problems,* 281–319.

Plant, M. A. (1986). *Drugs in perspective.* London: Hodder and Stoughton.

Population Services International. (2003). *Ivoirian soap-opera makes AIDS the talk of the town and wins FESPACO Film Festival award.* Retrieved August 20, 2003, from http://www.psi.org/resources/pubs/cotesoap.html.

The Portman Group. (2003). *2f3m4 Campaign.* Retrieved August 21, 2003, from http://www.portman-group.org.uk/campaigns/50.asp.

Rothman, K. J. (1993). Conflict of interest: The new McCarthyism in science. *Journal of the American Medical Association, 69,* 2782–2784.

Royal College of Obstetricians and Gynaecologists (RCOG). (1999). *Alcohol consumption in pregnancy* (RCOG Guideline No. 9). London: Author.

Shrader-Frechette, K. S. (1995). Evaluating the expertise of experts. *Risk, 6,* 115.

Smith-Warner, S. A., Spiegelman, D., Yaun, S. S., van den Brandt, P. A., Folsom, A. R., Goldbohm, R. A., et al. (1998). Alcohol and breast cancer in women: A pooled analysis of cohort studies. *Journal of the American Medical Association, 279,* 535–540.

Spadaro, R. (2003). *Eurobarometer 58.0. European Union citizens and sources of information about health.* European Opinion Research Group. Written for European Commission Health Consumer Protection Directorate-General (DG-SANCO). Retrieved August 19, 2003, from http://europa.eu.int/comm/public_opinion/archives/eb/ebs_179_en.pdf.

Streissguth, A. P., & O'Malley, K. (2000). Neuropsychiatric implications and long-term consequences of fetal alcohol spectrum disorders. *Seminars in Clinical Neuropsychiatry, 5,* 177–190.

Taig, T. (1999). Benchmarking in governments: Case studies and principles. In P. Bennet & K. Calman (Eds.), *Risk communication and public health* (pp. 117–132). New York: Oxford University Press.

United Nations Educational, Scientific and Cultural Organization. (2003). *Adolescent reproductive and sexual health: Advocacy and IEC strategies.* Retrieved October 15, 2003, from http://www.unescobkk.org/ips/arh-web/demographics/bangledesh/cfm.

Viljoen, D. (1999). Fetal alcohol syndrome. *South African Medical Journal, 89,* 958–960.

Warren, K. R., Calhoun, F. J., May, P. A., Viljoen, D. L., Li, T. K., Tanaka, H., et al. (2001). Fetal alcohol syndrome: An international perspective. *Alcoholism: Clinical and Experimental Research, 25,* 202S–206S.

Willis, J., & Okunade, A. A. (1997). *Reporting on risks: The practices and ethics of health and safety communication.* Westport, CT: Praeger.

The World Bank/International Bank for Reconstruction and Development (2000). *World development report 2000/2001: Attacking poverty.* New York: Oxford University Press.

Zunino, H., Litvak, J., & Israel, Y. (1998). Public and private partners in prevention and research: The case of the College of Pharmacy, University of Chile. In M. Grant & J. Litvak (Eds.), *Drinking patterns and their consequences* (pp. 282–285). Washington, DC: Taylor & Francis.

Chapter 5

To Do or Not to Do:
Risk Decisions

"Making decisions is like speaking prose—people do it all the time, knowingly or unknowingly."

Kahneman & Tversky, 2000, p. 1

Managing risk takes place on a number of levels. Whereas government agencies devise strategies and regulations to address potential harms, individuals
make daily decisions about how to manage the risk of driving a car or eating an
undercooked hamburger. Because nearly everything in life involves some risk,
these decisions require accepting some possibility of harm in order to achieve
benefits. The great uncertainty about the probabilities of harm resulting from
various behaviors means, "Evaluating risk requires interpretive judgment in the
face of technical uncertainty and scientific disagreement" (Nelkin, 1989, p. 95).

Dealing with risk is a matter of day-to-day decision making. On a personal level, managing risk doesn't necessarily mean reducing it. For example, enjoying risky sports doesn't minimize risk, but incorporates it into the
enjoyment of life. In some cases, society has no need to intervene; but when
a risky decision can hurt other people, intervention may be necessary
(British Medical Association, 1987).

This chapter focuses on how individuals use information about risks and
benefits to make decisions about their behavior. It briefly traces the history
of decision theory and examines how its concepts are used in contemporary
models of health behaviors. Next, it looks at some of the difficulties involved
in making decisions about health behavior, including the trade-offs of risks
and benefits and the effects of framing on health decisions. Finally, we apply
these models to decisions about alcohol consumption.

HISTORY OF DECISION THEORY

Analyses of risk, risky decisions, and decisions made with uncertainty are centuries old (Bernstein, 1996; Kammen & Hassenzahl, 1999). The beginnings of decision analysis can be seen as early as the 3rd century in Arnobius of Sicca's belief in God argument in *The Case against the Pagans*:

> Since, then, it is the nature of things which are still in the future that they cannot be grasped and understood by the touch of anticipation, is it not better reasoning that, of two alternatives which are both uncertain and hang in doubtful suspense, we should believe the one which affords some hopes rather than the one which offers none at all? In the former case there is no danger [if] what is said to be in the future proves vain and idle; and in the latter there is the greatest loss, specifically the loss of salvation, if when the time has come, it be made patent that there was no deceit (Arnobius of Sicca, Trans. 1949).

Arnobius thus argues that believing in God causes no harm if God does not actually exist, but affords hope of eternal life if God does exist; in this argument, one option (believing in God) is clearly superior to other alternatives (Kammen & Hassenzahl, 1999).

The birth of decision analysis is usually ascribed to the 17th-century philosopher Blaise Pascal, who put forward his famous Wager. In the notes for his book *Pensées* (1669/1910), Pascal reasoned that one cannot decide whether to believe in God ("God is, or He is not. Which way should we incline? Reason cannot answer."), but that one *can* decide how to live one's life—as if God exists, or as if God does not exist (Hájek, 2001). The question is framed in terms of a game of chance in which a person who leads a holy life is betting that God exists and a person who leads an unholy life wagers that there is no God. The way to choose how to live is to consider the outcomes of each choice, as listed in Table 5.1.

According to the Wager, the best way to win is by leading a holy life. If there is no God, you can live a good or a bad life without consequences; but if God does exist, living a holy life saves you from the eternal damnation suffered by the unholy. Heaven is clearly better than Hell; therefore, "To put it crudely, we should wager that God exists because it is the *best bet*" (Hájek, 2001).

TABLE 5.1

Choices	Possible Truths	
	God Does Not Exist	**God Exists**
Live a holy life	Nothing	Eternal life
Live an unholy life	Nothing	Damnation

Source: From Hájek, A. (2001) Pascal's wager. In E. Zalta (Ed.), *The standard encyclopedia of philosophy.* http://plato.stanford.edu/archives/win2001/entries/pascal-wager. Reprinted with author's permission.

Pascal's Wager is the first explicit example of principles of decision theory, or the theory of deciding what to do when the outcome is uncertain (Hacking, 1975; Hájek, 2001). In the Wager, the emphasis is on the severity of potential consequences of the decision (salvation or damnation), with no mention of the probability of the alternatives (God exists or does not). But Pascal also noted, "Fear of harm ought to be proportional not merely to the gravity of the harm, but also to the probability of the event" (Bernstein, 1996). That is, consequences can be either good or bad (or gradations in between) and can have varying probabilities (from nearly impossible to almost certain). The Wager represents the first expression of the concept of *utility,* which underlies theories of risk taking and decision making.

Utility was defined by Jeremy Bentham in the 18th century as ". . . that property in any object, whereby it tends to produce benefit, advantage, pleasure, good, or happiness . . . when the tendency it has to augment the happiness of the community is greater than any it has to diminish it" (Bernstein, 1996, p. 189). The utility of an item, a behavior, or a choice comprises both the probability of the potential consequences and the desirability of those outcomes. The highest utility is obtained when a consequence is very likely and very good; such a consequence (e.g., easing a headache with pain medication) is the most likely to "augment one's happiness." Consequences that are very unlikely but very good, such as winning the lottery, have relatively low utility simply because they are so unlikely to happen. In making decisions, we try to maximize expected utility by considering the probability and desirability of the potential consequences of the decision.

These basic principles—potential outcomes, the consequences of those outcomes, their probability, and their desirability—form the foundation of rational decision theory. In this view, people make decisions by totaling up the potential consequences of each alternative and choosing the alternative that maximizes utility. Decisions can be represented as a payoff matrix similar to the illustration of Pascal's Wager. Slovic, Kunreither, and White (2000, p. 3) give a simple illustration for a traveler in Table 5.2. The rows and columns contain the alternative selections and possible states of nature, and the cells contain the consequences that will result from each combination.

TABLE 5.2

	State of Nature	
Alternatives	**Sun**	**Rain**
Carry umbrella	stay dry carrying umbrella	stay dry carrying umbrella
Leave umbrella	dry and unburdened	wet and unburdened

Source: In P. Slovic et al. "Decision, Processes, Rationality, and Adjustment to Natural Hazards," from G. White *Natural Hazards: Local, National, Global.* Copyright 1974. Used by permission of Oxford University Press, Inc.

In most cases, it is not possible to arrive at a decision that will turn out to be the best, given any actual state of nature. Instead, when making a decision, we choose what we perceive to be the "best bet," which maximizes the utility of the decision. Thus, the combination of the best things offset by the fewest bad things is the best decision (Slovic, Kunreither, & White, 2000).

BEYOND A RATIONAL MODEL OF DECISION MAKING

When making real-life decisions, much of our information on potential outcomes is subjective. For example, suppose we are trying to decide whether to buy a house located near a flood plain. The probability of a flood during our lifetime is unknown, and, as we saw in Chapter 3, even expert estimates can be unreliable. Furthermore, the desirability (or undesirability) of the potential consequences of the decision is subjective: Some people are more terrified of floods than others are. Therefore, different people will have different utilities for the same outcome. For these reasons, we use the term *subjective expected utility* to refer to the perceived utility of the different outcomes when people make decisions about uncertain outcomes.

Another problematic aspect of rational decision theory is the practical problem of enumerating and rating all the subjective probabilities and values of various outcomes. For most decisions, numerous possible outcomes must be considered. For example, when deciding which apartment to rent or which house to buy, we consider location, price, size, parking, landscaping, schools, and several other factors. To make a rational decision, we would need to know ahead of time all possible outcomes, the probabilities for these outcomes, and the payoffs for all these outcomes. The computation of the utility of the decision quickly becomes extremely complex (Slovic et al., 2000).

The rational model of decision making is a normative model, which sets out the way that things should be, instead of a descriptive model of how things are really done. These decision-making models grew out of logical analyses of games of chance, instead of psychological analyses of people's actual notions of risk and value (Tversky & Kahneman, 2000). The idea that people use their mental prowess to choose rationally is intuitively appealing but easy to refute, given numerous examples of illogical decisions made by humans. Research in cognitive psychology and information processing demonstrates that human perceptual and intellectual processes are limited, and these cognitive limitations require simplified models of decision making (Slovic, Fischhoff, & Lichtenstein, 2000a). In reality, we humans don't have the time or ability to do the calculations required for rational decisions; instead, we have limited knowledge of decision alternatives and are uncertain about the possible outcomes.

Simplifying the Decision: "Satisficing" and Heuristics

A leading critic of the concept of utility maximization, economist Herbert Simon, proposed that rational decision models do not adequately describe real-life decisions. Simon argued that because of uncertainty about the future and the cognitive cost of acquiring information, we are unable to make fully rational decisions. Simon's theory of *bounded rationality* proposed that decision makers use a simplified model of decision making in which the key principle is not utility maximization but *satisficing,* or making do with a satisfactory (but not optimal) result. In this view, people don't think in probabilities and don't evaluate utilities to compare alternatives. Instead, they proceed by trial and error to produce a satisfactory result, and modify plans that fall short until they reach a satisfactory outcome (Slovic et al., 2000a). For example, a study of field commanders at fire scenes found just this pattern (Klein, 1998). The commanders did a quick mental run-through of the first reasonable plan that they conceived. If they discovered problems with that plan, they rejected it and looked for another, until they arrived at a plan with no foreseeable difficulties: "They don't need the best solution. They just need the one that works" (Breen, 2000b).

When dealing with tasks involving probabilities, people generally violate the principles of rational decision making. Instead, as noted in Chapter 1, they use simplification strategies called heuristics, or rules of thumb, to make decisions (Kahneman & Tversky, 2000). Although these strategies can lead to reasonable judgments, they often result in decisions that are biased in predictable ways (Slovic et al., 2000a). An extensive body of research has highlighted the errors that both experts and nonexperts experience when making judgments involving uncertain scenarios (Gilovich, Griffin, & Kahneman, 2002; Kahneman, Slovic, & Tversky, 1982; Tversky & Kahneman, 1974). For example, as we saw in Chapter 1 on risk perception, people tend to rely on ease of recall, or availability, to estimate probabilities. This means that very recent or vivid examples are viewed as more likely to happen. Other biases spring from the tendency to be more sensitive to potential loss than to potential gain, to prefer certainty to chance, and to discount small probabilities (Jeffery, 1989; Kahneman & Tversky, 1984).

This "heuristics and biases" approach assumes that human reasoning is error-prone by its very nature, and that our thought processes lead us to judgments that are demonstrably incorrect (the correct answer being the one arrived at by optimal mathematical formulas). Although this approach is influential in cognitive psychology, controversy exists regarding how bad humans really are at probabilistic information processing (Bower, 1996; Gigerenzer, 2000; Gilovich & Griffin, 2002; Sedlmeier, 1999) and about the relevance of these biases to real-world decisions (Cohen, 1993; Orasanu & Connolly, 1993).

A focus on naturalistic decision making questions the actual impact of cognitive biases when making real-world decisions. In this approach, people use strategies that effectively make use of their knowledge, revising and improving these strategies in changing environments (Klein, 1998; Klein, Orasanu, Calderwood, & Zsambok, 1993). The resulting performance is usually adequate. These strategies are qualitatively different from those identified in laboratory studies of information processing and are judged not in terms of their discrepancy from a "rational" outcome but by the functions they serve. Even decision processes that are formally inconsistent with probability theory can lead to useful outcomes when they embody the real-world knowledge of the decision makers (Cohen, 1993).

Risk as Feelings: Intuitive Decision Making

As most of us can attest, rational analysis is only part of what goes into making a decision. We approach many decisions from two different points of view: One is intuitive, automatic, and experiential; the other is analytic and rational (Epstein, 1994). In Chapter 1, we saw that affect, an automatic positive or negative evaluative feeling, can guide perceptions of risk and benefit. Moreover, these affective reactions can also guide subsequent decisions: "We sometimes delude ourselves that we proceed in a rational manner and weigh all the pros and cons of the various alternatives. But this is probably seldom the actual case. Quite often, 'I decided in favor of X' is no more than 'I liked X' " (Zajonc, 1980, p.155).

We often think of emotions as interfering with reason, but this intuitive process is an important component of how we navigate everyday life. "It was the experiential system, after all, that enabled human beings to survive during their long period of evolution. Long before there was probability theory, risk assessment, and decision analysis, there were intuition, instinct, and gut feeling to tell us whether an animal was safe to approach or the water was safe to drink" (Slovic, Finucane, Peters, & MacGregor, 2004). These fast and instinctive reactions serve as a mental shortcut that enables us to make judgments quickly and automatically in situations that would otherwise be too complex (Schwarz, 1988, 2002; Slovic et al., 2004).

Although this intuitive process often serves us well, it can mislead us in at least two ways (Slovic et al., in press; Slovic, Finucane, Peters, & MacGregor, 2002). First, those who wish to influence our behavior can sway our emotions. For example, advertisers are acutely aware of the influence of affect on decisions, and many advertising campaigns are almost solely affect-based. The pairing of cigarettes with images of rugged cowboys or a clean bathroom with the love and approval of one's family reflect the conviction that appealing to emotions can influence purchasing decisions. Similarly, public service announcements and charity appeals are nearly always laced with emotion.

Second, the inherent biases of the experiential system can lead to faulty judgments. Stalin's famous aphorism "A single death is a tragedy; a million deaths a statistic" exemplifies our tendency to be more emotionally affected by a single small change in our environment (the difference between 0 deaths and 1 death) than by changes of greater magnitude (the difference between 500 and 600 deaths) (Slovic et al., 2004). Other failures of affective judgment result from our inability to predict how we will feel in the future, especially when we are under the sway of drives such as hunger, thirst, or craving. In these situations, our emotions of the moment influence our behavior more than anticipated emotions (Loewenstein, 1999). For example, it is easier for the dieter tempted by chocolate to imagine its lovely taste than it is to imagine the guilt that might arise in the future from overindulgence in the present.

Analytic and experiential modes of decision making are constantly interacting. In fact, affect is a component of rational models of decision making, which incorporate decision makers' beliefs about whether alternative consequences are good or bad. Affect thus enables us to think rationally by its ability to "lubricate reason" (Slovic et al., in press). Reliance on emotions to make decisions can lead us to success when our "gut reaction" proves correct. However, when we overreact to frightening consequences, such as terrorism or shark attacks, analytic thinking can give us perspective on the likelihood of such consequences.

DECISIONS ABOUT HEALTH BEHAVIOR

The major principles of utility—probability of possible outcomes and desirability of those outcomes—are central to most theories of health behavior. Many models have been proposed to explain how people adopt health-protective

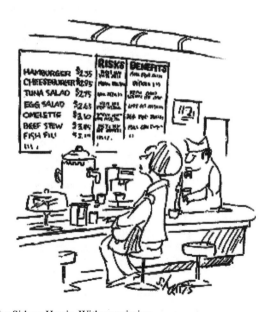

Copyright 2004 by Sidney Harris. With permission.

behavior or abandon behavior that is harmful to health (Weinstein, 1993). These theories assume that people are motivated toward self-protection when they anticipate a negative outcome and desire to reduce its impact. The motivation is driven primarily by two factors: the perceived severity of the potential outcome and the perceived likelihood that the outcome will occur (also called perceived vulnerability or perceived susceptibility). For example, a smoker's motivation to quit smoking will be driven by her beliefs about how likely she is to experience bad things as a result of smoking (e.g., contract smoking-related diseases, spend too much money, or have yellow teeth) and her perceptions of how unpleasant each of these consequences would be.

The motivation to adopt a health-protective behavior arises from the individual's expectation that such an action will reduce either the likelihood of harm or its severity. At the same time, the models assume that costs, as well as benefits, are involved in adopting health-protective behavior, and these costs must be weighed against the expected benefits in risk reduction that accrue from behavior change (Weinstein, 1993). For example, the costs of quitting smoking include loss of satisfaction from smoking, experiencing cravings, potential weight gain, and so on. To the extent that the benefits of quitting smoking outweigh the costs, the motivation to quit outweighs the motivation to continue smoking. Thus, the premise of these models is that people estimate the seriousness of the risk or symptoms, evaluate the costs and benefits of action, and choose the course that maximizes expected outcome (Cleary, 1987). "The view of individuals as decision makers striving to weigh the potential costs of taking a precaution against the benefits that may be received is the basis for the most widespread model of self-protective behavior" (Weinstein, 1987, p. 325).

So far, the models of health behavior we have discussed are simply a restatement of utility theory, in which people act to maximize good outcomes and minimize bad outcomes. However, these models also incorporate other variables that affect behavior, including:

- The perceived *effectiveness* of the precaution (Janz & Becker, 1984). Will adopting the behavior bring about the expected outcome. If, for example, the smoker believes that quitting smoking will not reduce her chances of illness, then there is no particular reason to stop.
- *Self-efficacy,* or the individual's expected ability to carry out the behavior change (Rogers, 1983): If the smoker thinks that she simply won't be successful in quitting, her motivation to do so is decreased.
- Perceived *social norms* (i.e., What do other people important to you think about your behavior [(Ajzen & Fishbein, 1980]?): An adolescent who smokes to fit in with friends may think her friends wouldn't like it if she quit. If so, she is less likely to stop.

Weinstein (1993) notes that these models are oversimplified in that they focus on just one decision event: whether or not to act. Adopting health behaviors, however, is more complex than that. The process incorporates several distinct steps that must be explained:

1. How people first come to consider a problem as requiring their attention.
2. What makes people decide they should act.
3. What kinds of barriers intervene between the decision to act and actually doing something ("the best-laid plans . . . "). Furthermore, different factors may be involved in initiating a behavior and maintaining that behavior (Cleary, 1987).

When we examine health behaviors from a utility point of view, we can see several reasons why people frequently fail to adopt health protective behaviors:

• Information on complicated risks is often unknown or undependable (Weinstein, 1987). Most people simply do not know the actual probabilities of contracting HIV from unprotected sex, getting diabetes as the result of a sedentary lifestyle, or harming their hearts through lack of exercise. Moreover, as discussed in Chapter 1, perception of risk is affected by various cognitive biases.
• It is difficult to know to what extent a health-protective action will reduce risk (Cleary, 1987). If I exercise daily, how much does that reduce my risk of coronary disease in the future?
• Even when people have a fairly good idea that their behaviors are harmful, they may think that they have plenty of time to change it before it becomes *too* harmful. For example, although young smokers are well aware of the risks of smoking, to the extent that they even overestimate the risks of a smoker getting lung cancer, they also believe that smoking for only a few years poses negligible risk. Moreover, they severely underestimate the difficulty of quitting smoking. As a result, young smokers believe themselves to be at little risk from smoking because they expect to stop smoking before any damage to their health occurs (Slovic, 2001).
• Although perceived costs and benefits are important in motivating behavior, people tend to focus disproportionately on short-term instead of long-term outcomes. Whereas future harm is only a possibility, the costs of implementing behavior change in the present, be it using a condom or eating fewer calories, are harder to accept (Jeffery, 1989; Weinstein, 1987).
• Many so-called "health behaviors" serve functions unrelated to health, and the motivation to avoid harm is only one of many motives inherent in most health-related situations (Cleary, 1987). For example, using condoms can reduce HIV transmission, but their use is also entangled with other motives reflecting desire, sexual satisfaction, and trust. For some behaviors, including drinking, drugs, and sex, the desire to avoid risk may be less powerful than positive motivations such as pleasure and pleasing others (Weinstein, 1989).

• Deciding what to do to protect one's health is difficult, given that one can do so in many ways (Cleary, 1987). For example, if one wants to lower cholesterol, a number of alternatives are available, including exercise, weight loss, and medications; to avoid contracting HIV, one could stop having sex altogether, use condoms consistently, or have sex only with partners who have tested negative for HIV.

In summary, utility-based models of health-preventive behavior don't tell the whole story. Many health behaviors are not based on explicit decision-making processes; instead, they might reflect habit, carelessness, or the emotions of the present, instead of consideration of the future. Even when people do attempt to behave rationally, it's difficult to estimate risk and the effects of behavior on lowering that risk. Because health behaviors do not occur in isolation, it is important to consider social contexts and the meaning of health behaviors in serving other functions.

Trade-Offs of Risks and Benefits

One of the paradoxes of risk reduction is that reducing one risk may result in an increase in another (Keeney, 1994). Many kinds of countervailing risks are commonly known as "side effects" (i.e., in medicine), "collateral damage" (i.e., in military tactics), or "unintended consequences" (i.e., in public policy) (Graham & Wiener, 1995, p. 2). Weighing these risks poses a problem for anyone trying to figure out how to optimize health; making health decisions can become very complex when one has to focus on many potential outcomes (National Research Council, 1996).

Examples of these trade-offs abound:

• Drinking alcohol in moderation may be, in some cases, good for the heart but bad for other systems.
• Now that tourists can be vaccinated against diseases that aren't present in their home countries, they can travel to exotic parts of the world. This travel exposes them to yet more diseases and dangers (Adams, 1999).
• Taking aspirin for a headache may upset your stomach.
• The Davy lamp (invented in 1816 by Sir Humphry Davy) was designed to operate at a temperature below that required to ignite methane, thus preventing mine explosions. Miners could also use the Davy lamp as a crude test for the presence of flammable gases, which make the lamp burn with a blue tinge, or for carbon dioxide, which extinguishes the lamp. This life-saving invention made it possible for miners to go farther into methane-rich areas of the mines, which increased mining productivity but also increased explosions and fatalities (Adams, 1999).
• Tamoxifen prevents recurrence of breast cancer, but may increase risk for endometrial cancer (Fisher et al., 1998).

- Spraying hot water to clean the oil from the site of an oil tanker spill in Prince William Sound, Alaska, in 1989 reduced the risk to birds and mammals, but killed smaller marine organisms that lived on and under the beach (Graham & Wiener, 1995).
- Hospital care for trauma and illnesses increases the risk of hospital-acquired infections.
- Repeated scrubbing of public monuments removes dirt and graffiti, but may cause serious crumbling of the stone (Graham & Wiener, 1995).
- Prohibition of alcohol in the U.S. during the 1920s and 1930s reduced the incidence of liver cirrhosis but opened up markets for illegal distribution.
- Removing asbestos from homes and schools to protect residents and students increases the risk of contracting lung diseases for those removing the asbestos.

We weigh one risk against other risks all the time as we decide, for instance, whether to drive or fly, or to take aspirin or acetominophen. The key factors in making these judgments include (Graham & Wiener, 1995):

- *The magnitude or relative probabilities of risks.* The target risk and countervailing risk often differ in magnitude or in the probability that they will occur. If so, we can weigh the two probabilities in making decisions. For example, the probability of illness from pesticides used in growing fruits and vegetables is smaller than the estimated probability that eating fruits and vegetables helps to prevent heart disease, stroke, and certain kinds of cancer.
- *The certainty of the risk estimates.* Although uncertainty always exists in risk estimates, some estimates are supported by science, while others are based on speculation.
- *The type of adverse outcome.* For some behaviors, the potential adverse outcomes may be sufficiently similar that they can be compared to form an idea of "net risk." For example, when deciding whether to eat fish for dinner, we might compare the increased risk of cancer (from contaminants found in fish) with the decreased risk of heart disease (from beneficial fatty acids). For other behaviors, however, the different types of outcomes can be particularly difficult to compare: Is death from cancer, accident, and heart disease really equivalent? As discussed in Chapter 1, various risk outcomes carry differing amounts of subjective "dread," and, indeed, some research has shown that people view avoiding death from cancer as about twice as desirable as avoiding sudden accidental death (Tolley, Kenkel, & Fabian, 1994).
- *Whether the risks are immediate or delayed.* Sometimes, the timing of the target risk and the countervailing risk differ. For example, we might reduce risk of death in an automobile accident by wearing seat belts, driving during the daytime, and driving carefully. By keeping ourselves alive in the short term, however, we increase our risk of dying of a chronic disease, such as cancer, later in life. Should we try to reduce immediate risks at the expense of future risks?

The Role of Framing in Health Decisions

In 1995, the British Committee on the Safety of Medicines issued a warning about a new type of oral contraceptive, stating that the new pill was twice as likely as the older formula to cause potentially fatal blood clots. As a result, many women stopped taking the new pill, leading to an estimated 8,000 extra abortions and an unknown number of unplanned pregnancies. It then emerged that this doubling of risk represented an increase in the death rate from 3 per million to 6 per million—a risk well below the mortality from abortions and pregnancies. The government's chief medical officer later admitted that the assessment should have been put into some sort of context (Adams, 1999; Matthews, 1998).

These events illustrate the effect of *framing*, or presenting logically equivalent information in different ways. In its warning to British women, the Committee chose to frame the information in terms of relative risk: the risk of blood clots among women taking the new pill divided by the risk among women taking older pills (6 per million/3 per million = 2, or twice the risk). The same information could be presented as the difference in absolute risk, which in this case was .0000003 (.0000006 − .0000003). Although no one knows what the response of British women would have been to such a warning, research on the effects of framing suggests that it would have been much less extreme.

When calculating results from clinical trials or other kinds of epidemiologic studies, several measures of risk can be used, all of which express the same information but in different ways. To illustrate, consider the results of a study of the effects of antihypertensive medication on subsequent stroke (Collins et al., 1990). The statistics that can be calculated from these data include:

Probability of stroke: the number of people in a group who suffered a stroke, divided by the total number of people in that group;

Relative risk: the probability of stroke in the drug group, divided by the probability of stroke in the no-drug group;

Relative risk reduction: 1 minus the relative risk, multiplied by 100; for example, if the relative risk is .8, the relative risk reduction is 20%;

Risk difference: the probability of stroke in the drug group minus the probability of stroke in the no-drug group;

Number needed to treat: 1 divided by the risk difference; this number represents the number of people that would need to be treated to prevent one stroke (adapted from Sackett & Cook, 1994).

As illustrated in Table 5.3, patients with moderate to severe hypertension were less likely to suffer a stroke after 5 years if they were treated with antihypertensive medication. In terms of a relative risk reduction, drug treatment reduced stroke by 40%, representing a risk difference of .08 (.20 probability of stroke with no drugs, minus .12 probability of stroke with

TABLE 5.3

	Number of strokes per 15,000 patients after 5 years	Probability of stroke	Relative risk	Relative risk reduction	Risk difference	Number needed to treat
Patients with moderate to severe hypertension						
No drug	3000	.20	—	—	—	—
Drug	1800	.12	.6	40%	.08	13

drugs). Thirteen people with moderate to severe hypertension would have to be treated in order to prevent one stroke (Sackett & Cook, 1994).

Now consider what happens among patients with less severe hypertension, whose risk of stroke is substantially lower (Table 5.4). The relative risk reduction attributed to the drug treatment is still 40%, but this represents a risk difference of only .006, and 167 patients would have to be treated in order to prevent one stroke. Thus, when overall susceptibility to stroke is high, a 40% relative risk reduction represents 8 strokes prevented for every 100 patients, but when susceptibility is low, the same relative risk reduction represents less than 1 stroke prevented for every 100 patients (Sackett & Cook, 1994).

Figure 5.1 depicts relative risk and risk differences in a hypothetical study of three different populations that vary in underlying risk of the outcome (Guyatt & Rennie, 2002, p. 352). When viewed as relative risk, the effect of the hypothetical treatment is the same for all the populations—a relative risk reduction of 33%. When viewed as a risk difference, however, the treatment effect varies greatly among the three groups. In a group that is initially at high risk (Population 1), the risk is reduced from 30% to 20%, a difference of 10%, while in a low-risk group (Population 3), the risk is only minimally reduced, from 3% to 2%.

TABLE 5.4

	Number of strokes per 15,000 patients after 5 years	Probability of stroke	Relative risk	Relative risk reduction	Risk difference	Number needed to treat
Patients with mild hypertension						
No drug	225	.015	—	—	—	—
Drug	135	.009	.6	40%	.006	167

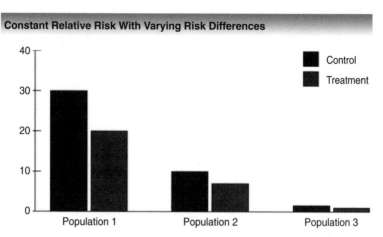

FIGURE 5.1. General and personal alcohol risk as function of amount of alcohol consumed per week (men & women). From *User's Guide to the Medical Literature: A Manual for Evidence-Based Clinical Practice*, Copyright 2002. Reprinted with permission of the American Medical Association.

Although relative risk reduction, risk difference, and number needed to treat are all correct and reflect the same information, they suggest different degrees of benefits and evoke different reactions. Relative risk reduction figures look quite impressive (Steiner, 1999). The larger numbers used to describe relative risk suggest higher benefits than do the smaller numbers that spell out risk difference. After all, a 40% risk reduction sounds much more impressive than a risk difference of 6/1000 (Gigerenzer, 2002).

This tendency to view the larger risk reduction percentages as conferring greater benefit can be exploited by organizations that want to emphasize the beneficial effects of a treatment. Pharmaceutical companies consistently use relative risk reduction in advertisements for medications (Skolbekken, 1998) and consumer information about the benefits of diet, treatment, or screening focuses on relative risk reductions instead of absolute differences (McCormack & Levine, 1993). To increase or decrease a patient's willingness to accept a medical treatment, physicians and drug companies can represent benefits of the treatment in terms of relative risk reductions and the risks in terms of absolute risk differences. For example, leaflets describing hormone therapy distributed in the offices of German gynecologists state that hormone therapy "protects women against colorectal cancer (by up to more than 50%). That is, women who receive hormone therapy develop colorectal cancer only half as often." The leaflet also states that hormone therapy is associated with a "minimal increase" in the lifetime incidence of breast cancer, from 60 in 1000 women to 66 in 1000 women: "That is, the risk may possibly increase by .6 percent (6 in 1000)." In this leaflet, the potential risks of hormone therapy are presented as absolute risk differences, which appear to be quite small, and the potential benefits of therapy are presented as relative risk reductions, which appear to be quite large (Gigerenzer, 2002).

Does the framing of a medical finding in terms of relative or absolute risk affect people's decisions about treatment? Studies of both physicians and patients suggest that it does. When physicians are presented with results of clinical trials framed as relative risk reductions, they express more enthusiasm for the treatment than when the results are presented as absolute risk differences. Physicians who see the relative risk numbers are also more likely to rate the treatment as effective and to express intentions to treat their patients accordingly (McGettigan, Sly, O'Connell, Hill, & Henry, 1999).

For interventions that show adverse treatment effects (i.e., the intervention resulted in poorer outcomes for those treated), physicians viewed the treatment more negatively if the results were presented as relative risks. For example, Swiss general practitioners and internists were given questionnaires that presented the results of the Helsinki Heart Study (Heinonen et al., 1994), a prevention trial that assessed the effectiveness of a lipid-lowering medication on the risk of heart attack in men with high cholesterol. Half of the questionnaires presented the results in terms of reduction in relative risk, and the other half presented results as absolute risk differences. Physicians were asked to rate the effectiveness of the lipid-lowering medication and to rate their likelihood of using the medication to treat high cholesterol in an otherwise healthy man. Physicians who received the absolute risk information rated the effectiveness of the medication as lower than did physicians who received relative risk reduction information and were less inclined to treat high cholesterol with the medication (Bucher, Weinbacher, & Gyr, 1994).

Patients, as well as physicians, are more impressed with relative risk than with absolute risk (Hux & Naylor, 1995; Malenka, Baron, Johansen, Wahrenberger, & Ross, 1993; Misselbrook & Armstrong, 2001). In a Canadian study that also used information from the Helsinki Heart Study, patients were given information about the effects of lipid-lowering medication on the risk of heart attack in terms of relative risk, absolute risk difference, and number needed to treat. To assess the perceptions of these different statistics, patients were presented with the information as if these numbers came from three different medications; they were also asked to decide whether they would be willing to take each medication. When the information was presented in terms of relative risk reduction (34% reduction in heart attacks), 88% of patients consented to therapy. When the absolute risk difference was presented (1.4% fewer patients had heart attacks), 42% consented. When number needed to treat was presented (71 persons needed to be treated for 5 years to prevent 1 heart attack), 31% consented to treatment (Hux & Naylor, 1995).

Procedures or treatments are also more likely to be viewed favorably by both physicians and patients if the potential consequences are presented in terms of good outcomes (e.g., percentage survival), instead of bad outcomes (e.g., percentage mortality) (Edwards, Elwyn, Covey, Matthews, & Pill, 2001; McGettigan et al., 1999). In a study of patients, physicians, and graduate students, subjects were asked to imagine that they had lung cancer and must choose between radiation therapy and surgery. Information about the potential outcomes of the two treatments was presented in terms of life or death (subjects were told that surgery resulted in either a 32% chance of death after a year, or a 68% chance of survival after a year). When the predicted outcome was presented in terms of survival, 72% chose surgery, but when the outcome was presented in terms of mortality, only 56% chose surgery. Thus, despite the fact that surgery entails the risk of death during treatment and radiation does not, the surgery option was seen as more attractive when the decision was framed in terms of life instead of death (McNeil, Pauker, Sox, & Tversky, 1982).

Furthermore, framing of outcomes in terms of lifetime probability, instead of the probability of a single event, can affect decisions. Slovic and colleagues (Slovic, Fischhoff, & Lichtenstein, 2000b) note that many people do not wear seat belts despite good evidence that they reduce death and injury from automobile accidents. Although people are aware of the effectiveness of seat belts, they may decline to wear them simply because the probability of an accident on any single automobile trip is so small: A fatal accident would be expected to occur in only 1 of every 3.5 million person-trips, and a disabling injury would be expected in 1 of every 100,000 person-trips. When we consider the cumulative probability of death or injury over 50 years of driving, however, the probabilities are substantial: a 1 in 100 chance of death and a 1 in 3 chance of a disabling injury. In one study, people were given information about crash risk either on a per-trip basis or within a lifetime perspective. Receiving the lifetime information led to more favorable attitudes toward the use of seat belts, more support for laws requiring seat belts, and more intentions to use seat belts in the future (Slovic, Fischhoff, & Lichtenstein, 1978).

Even the use of raw numbers instead of percentages can affect people's attitudes toward health decisions. Participants in a Swiss study were asked to imagine that they were suffering from a serious illness that would be fatal without medication, and that they were currently taking a medication (cost: $185) that reduced the probability of dying from the illness to .0006. They were then asked how much they would pay for a new medication that would reduce the probability of dying to .0003. When the probabilities of dying with the old and new medication were presented as .0006 and .0003, the subjects were willing to pay an average of $213 for the new medication—slightly more than the $185 for the current medication. But when the probabilities were cast in terms of frequencies instead of fractions (i.e., the medication would reduce risk from 600 to 300 in 1 million), the subjects were willing to pay substantially more for the new medication: $362. If the risks were described as extremely small (6 and 3 in 1 million), the difference in the acceptable payment for the old and new medications disappeared (Siegrist, 1997).

Research on framing of outcomes points to a tendency to be more accepting of health interventions when the results of those interventions are framed
in terms of potential benefits instead of potential risks, relative risk compared
with absolute risk, lifetime outcomes compared with single-event outcomes,
and frequencies compared with probabilities. The latter three scenarios may
reflect an individual's tendency to be more impressed with larger numbers,
irrespective of what the numbers represent. Relative risk seems larger than
absolute risk, cumulative probabilities are larger than single-event probabilities, and actual numbers representing small probabilities are easier to digest
than those small probabilities incorporating several decimal points.

Population vs. Individual Risk

When people make decisions about their own health behaviors, they want to be
armed with information that explains ways to reduce their individual risk for
negative outcomes. We receive such information in many ways: from physician
counseling, health reports in the media, and scientific sources (Rockhill, 2001).
This information, most of which comes from clinical studies, summarizes the
ways in which health behaviors relate to risk in populations. Unfortunately, risk
factors identified on the population level are poor predictors for individuals
(Rose, 1985). That is, on a population level, we might say that a particular risk
factor (e.g., smoking) increases the risk of lung cancer by a factor of 10, from a
.03% probability to a .3% probability. For each individual, however, the probability is either 1 (you contract lung cancer) or 0 (you don't).

On a population level, very small risks can make a big difference if they
are widespread and the population is large. For example, reducing cholesterol among men over 55 leads to an absolute risk reduction of about .02
(i.e., 2 in 100 men will avoid a heart attack as a result of the cholesterol
reduction). The other 98 would "eat differently every day for 40 years and
perhaps get nothing from it" (Rose, 1981, p. 1850) But because heart disease
is the most common cause of death in the U.S. and approximately 20% of the
population has high cholesterol levels, reducing cholesterol on a population
level would prevent thousands of deaths each year.

Thus, if a risk factor is related to a disease on the aggregate level, it does
not necessarily mean that an individual with that risk factor can prevent the
disease by eliminating the risk factor. As the previous example involving
cholesterol points out, the probabilities of risk reduction are such that out of
many people who modify their behavior with an eye to reducing their risk
(e.g., by taking a medication, submitting to a medical intervention, or increasing healthy behavior), only a few will benefit as a result. We can know
in advance neither whether a bad outcome will be prevented for an individual, nor can we know after the fact whether an intervention has prevented a
bad outcome. The benefits of treatment or risk reduction are realized by populations, not individuals (Rockhill, 2001; Steiner, 1999).

DECISIONS ABOUT ALCOHOL

As we have seen, models of decision making regarding health incorporate two central variables: perceived vulnerability (susceptibility) and perceived severity of outcomes. Most bad health outcomes—injury, disease, or premature death—are assumed undesirable. If utility models approximate health decisions, then it should follow that people who see themselves as likely to experience harm will drink less than those who see themselves as less likely to experience harm.

Chapter 1 discussed the fact that alcohol is associated with both perceived risk and benefit. How do these elements combine to influence drinking decisions? Is the perceived risk of alcohol consumption related to drinking? That is, does a high-risk perception keep people from drinking, and does a low-risk perception encourage drinking? Some research indicates that heavier drinkers perceive the risks of drinking, including the risks of drinking during pregnancy and driving while intoxicated, as less likely than do lighter drinkers (Agostinelli & Miller, 1994; Gonzalez & Haney, 1990; Greenfield & Rogers, 1999; Morris, Swasy, & Mazis, 1994; Stutts, Patterson, & Hunnicutt, 1997; Testa & Reifman, 1996). Most of the studies that show a negative correlation of alcohol consumption to risk perception have either failed to specify the risk target or have specified the risk not as alcohol consumption but as excessive consumption or illegal behavior, such as drunk driving (Sjöberg, 1998).

Given that heavier drinkers are, in reality, at greater risk for negative alcohol-related outcomes, the finding that heavier drinkers perceive lesser risk might have several different explanations:

- Consistent with utility-based models of health behavior, perceived vulnerability may motivate behavior: A perception of low risk from drinking leads to heavier drinking habits, and a perception of higher risk leads to lighter drinking habits.
- Heavier drinkers perceive lower risk because their drinking experience has shown them that bad things rarely happen to them. If they have not experienced problems from drinking, despite extensive drinking experience, they may be more likely to believe that problems won't occur in the future (Weinstein, 1989).
- The lower risk perception of heavier drinkers may reflect denial. Heavier drinkers might, on some level, be aware of their increased risk, but they are motivated to minimize these risks as a protective mechanism (Agostinelli & Miller, 1994).

Other studies, however, have demonstrated that heavier drinkers rate their likelihood of risk as greater than that of light drinkers (Wieczorek, Mirand, & Callahan, 1994; Wild & Cunningham, 2001; Wild, Hinson, Cunningham, & Bacchiochi, 2001). These perceptions are probably accurate, given that heavier drinkers report more harm from drinking (Room, Bondy, & Ferris, 1995). Thus, there is an "element of rationality" in risk perceptions about drinking

(Sjöberg, 1998), and these perceptions reflect awareness of actual risk status instead of denial. Despite these reasonable perceptions, heavier drinkers still manifest the optimistic bias discussed in Chapter 1: They perceive their own risk as lower than that of others.

For example, a Swedish survey asked respondents to rate their own risks from drinking, as well as risks for people in general. The more people drank, the more highly they rated their own risk, although the rated risk for people in general did not vary by alcohol consumption. As illustrated in Figure 5.2, however, people underestimated their own levels of risk, with only the heaviest drinkers rating their personal risks as equivalent to the risk for the population in general (Sjöberg, 1998).

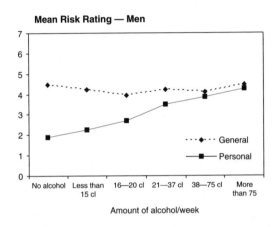

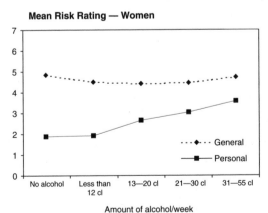

FIGURE 5.2. General and personal alcohol risk as function of amount of alcohol consumed per week (men & women). Adopted from Sjöberg, L. (1998). Risk perception of alcohol consumption. *Alcoholism: Clinical and Experimental Research, 22*(Suppl. 7), 277S–279S. Reprinted with permission from Lippincott, Williams & Wilkins.

Research on alcohol expectancies, as discussed in Chapter 1, might serve to illuminate the relationship of the perceived risks and benefits of drinking. From the viewpoint of expectancy, if people drink to achieve certain desirable consequences or to avoid undesirable ones, people with stronger positive expectancies should drink more, while those with stronger negative expectancies should drink less. The picture is not nearly this simple, however.

Some research findings demonstrate that heavier drinkers view negative effects as less likely to occur than do lighter drinkers (Mann, Chassin, & Sher, 1987; Roizen, 1983; Young & Knight, 1989), while other studies suggest that heavier drinkers view negative effects as more likely to occur than do lighter drinkers (Connors, O'Farrell, Cutter, & Thompson, 1987; Leigh, 1987, 1989; Stacy, Widaman, & Marlatt, 1990). The inconsistency of the relationship of negative expectancies to amount of drinking casts doubt on a utility model that says people drink because they expect the effects to be positive overall (Adams & McNeil, 1991). Clearly, heavy drinkers do expect—and experience—negative outcomes from drinking. So, why don't these negative expectancies lead to lighter drinking (McMahon & Jones, 1994)?

Negative effects are "swamped" by positive effects. As described in Chapter 1, people who expect negative consequences from drinking also expect positive consequences; however, for most drinkers, many potential negative effects, including effects on health, family life, and legal status, occur infrequently if at all. The possibility of negative outcomes may be "swamped" by the much more probable likelihood of pleasurable consequences. Thus, although people know that negative effects may occur from using alcohol, they may be more motivated by the positive effects that are more likely.

Negative effects are evaluated as not so bad. Labeling alcohol effects as "positive" or "negative" is problematic, given that effects that are desirable to some people may be undesirable for others. A striking example of this subjectivity comes from a study in which people were asked to list the positive and negative effects of alcohol (Leigh & Stacy, 1994). Whereas 14% of men and 5% of women listed increased sexuality as a positive consequence of drinking, 6% of men and 13% of women mentioned it as a negative consequence. Clearly, some alcohol effects are positive to some and negative to others.

Heavier drinkers tend to perceive alcohol effects less negatively than do lighter drinkers and nondrinkers (Cahalan & Room, 1974; Critchlow, 1987; Gustafson, 1991, 1993; Leigh, 1987, 1989; McCarty, Morrison, & Mills, 1983; Roizen, 1983). These perceptions may result from the norms of drinking situations. If heavy drinkers drink mostly with other heavy drinkers who are also experiencing negative consequences, they may accept these consequences as normal (McMahon & Jones, 1994). If bad outcomes are considered as not so bad, these outcomes may not effectively limit drinking.

Whether drinking has utility depends both on the probability of the consequences and the desirability of the consequences. Each of these characteristics varies among individuals. In the case of drinking, some may perceive certain consequences of alcohol consumption as highly likely to occur, while others may see their likelihood as relatively low; some may consider certain consequences as extremely desirable, while others may not. Thus, the relative "payoff" for drinking will vary greatly.

Positive effects are immediate and more likely to be learned. Many positive effects of alcohol are immediate, "feel-good" consequences, while many negative effects are delayed: by minutes (loss of coordination), days (loss of job), or years (loss of liver function). In humans, alcohol effects often demonstrate a biphasic pattern in which an initial increase in excitation, arousal, and euphoria is followed by depression and dysphoria (Mello, 1968). These differing effects may result from rising and falling levels of blood alcohol (Jones & Vega, 1972).

The delay between drinking and bad consequences means that the association of the two is less likely to be learned. For example, dog owners know that in order to teach a puppy not to chew on shoes, punishment for chewing must be applied immediately so that the puppy associates the punishment with the chewing (and not with something else that has happened in between). Human learning is similar: If negative effects of drinking are delayed relative to positive effects, they are less likely to be associated with alcohol. The relative importance of desirable and undesirable consequences in drinking motivation might then be a function of the immediacy of the consequence. For drinkers, the pleasurable, reinforcing "ups" are more immediate and thus may have a greater impact on learning about drinking and its effects than the more delayed "downs." A drinking episode might end badly, but its pleasurable beginnings are more powerful motivators (Marlatt, 1987; Stacy & Widaman, 1987).

In addition, some severe negative consequences of drinking, including accidents and long-term physical damage, are never experienced by most drinkers and thus are not learned by direct experience. Drinkers who have not experienced serious consequences will perceive them as unlikely to occur in the future, and these consequences may not figure strongly in drinking decisions. Stacy (1986) and Stacy and Widaman (1987) suggest that "beliefs about positive outcomes are more likely to be based on direct experience than are beliefs about negative outcomes, possibly leading to a bias in 'retrievability' favoring positive outcomes" (Stacy & Widaman, 1987). Expectancies that are more easily retrievable are viewed as more probable (Tversky & Kahneman, 1974) and thus may more strongly affect intentions to drink.

Positive and Negative Expectancies: Social Drinkers vs. Problem Drinkers

Relationships between positive expectancies, negative expectancies, and drinking may well differ during drinking careers. McMahon, Jones, and

O'Donnell (1994) argue that among social drinkers, expectancies of negative consequences should increase with increasing consumption: As social drinkers drink more heavily, they experience more negative consequences and thus expect more negative consequences in the future. At some point, however, when drinking reaches problematic levels, negative expectancy begins to exert stronger influence on drinking decisions. Clearly, it is expectations of negative consequences that lead heavy drinkers to moderate their drinking or seek treatment.

In a series of studies of alcohol-dependent clients in treatment, Jones and McMahon found that positive expectancy had little or no relationship to treatment outcome, but that clients with stronger expectations of negative consequences were less likely to relapse within 3 months of treatment and remained abstinent longer (Jones & McMahon, 1994a, 1994b, 1996a, 1996b; McMahon & Jones, 1996). Moreover, the expectancies most strongly related to treatment outcome were expectancies of longer-term consequences of continued drinking, such as health effects, instead of consequences that happen right after drinking (e.g., unpleasant social behavior) or the next day (e.g., a hangover). McMahon et al. (1994) argue that expectancies of delayed effects are more important in motivating changes in drinking because problem drinkers tend to misperceive the more immediate negative consequences of drinking and underestimate their negative nature.

It is not yet clear whether risk perceptions or expectancies are a result of alcohol consumption or one of its causes (Sjöberg, 1998). Although utility-based models predict that risk perceptions should motivate behavior, some research suggests that behavior itself affects risk perceptions. Most research studies cannot distinguish between the chicken and the egg: Relationships between risk perception and risk behaviors might reflect motivations or accuracy of risk perceptions, with no way to differentiate these possibilities (Weinstein & Nicolich, 1993). Longitudinal research, in which changes in risk perceptions and changes in drinking patterns are tracked over time, can shed light on the ways in which motivational and experiential factors relate to each other over time (Aas, Leigh, Anderssen, & Jakobsen, 1998).

SUMMARY

> ". . . a person has only one decision to make in his whole life. He must, namely, decide how to live, and this he might in principle do once and for all."

> *Savage, 1954, p. 83*

Deciding how to live can be a matter of psychology, philosophy, or religion. As we have seen in this chapter, although we may like to believe that we make decisions carefully, by weighing positives and negatives, our daily decisions are often driven by habit, intuition, or emotions. Some decisions are agonizing (Which university should I attend? Which job offer should I accept?); some are not (Which tie goes with this shirt?). When it comes to decisions about health, we are influenced by information—both its content and the way in which it is presented. We read the paper or watch television news, and we try to synthesize what we find out about the risks and benefits of things we do every day (e.g., driving on the roads or drinking chemically treated water) as well as things that most of us never experience (e.g., living near a chemical spill).

Decisions about drinking, a regular activity for many, depend not only on our beliefs about its consequences but the social context in which they occur. Balancing the positive and negative outcomes of drinking is only part of what goes into drinking decisions. As we discussed in other chapters, the meaning and acceptability of different consequences of drinking vary across cultures, genders, and age groups.

Decisions about risk are individual decisions, and the choices people make vary substantially. Because of this variation in risk–benefit calculations and emotional responses, some people do things that others would never even consider. Scuba divers who explore underwater cave systems are often viewed as extreme risk takers, but cave diver Wes Skiles explains that these divers manage the risk with meticulous planning, multiple backup systems, and sophisticated equipment. "We're comfortable living inside of a bubble that would scare the hell out of most people. So when you ask, 'Are you going to do anything dangerous?' what do you want to hear? From us, the answer is no. We're not doing anything dangerous. But evaluated by you, we're freaking out of our minds" (Breen, 2000a).

REFERENCES

Aas, H., Leigh, B. C., Anderssen, N., & Jakobsen, R. (1998). Two-year longitudinal study of alcohol expectancies and drinking among Norwegian adolescents. *Addiction, 93,* 373–384.

Adams, J. (1999). *Cars, cholera, and cows: The management of risk and uncertainty.* Washington, DC: Cato Institute.

Adams, S. L., & McNeil, D. W. (1991). Negative alcohol expectancies reconsidered. *Psychology of Addictive Behaviors, 5*(1), 9–14.

Agostinelli, G., & Miller, W. R. (1994). Drinking and thinking: How does personal drinking affect judgments of prevalence and risk? *Journal of Studies on Alcohol, 55*(3), 327–337.

Ajzen, I., & Fishbein, M. (1980). *Understanding attitudes and predicting behavior.* Englewood Cliffs, NJ: Prentice Hall.

Arnobius of Sicca. (1949). *The case against the pagans* (G. E. McCracken, Trans., Vol. 7). New York: Paulist Press. (Original work published circa 302)

Bernstein, P. L. (1996). *Against the gods: The remarkable story of risk.* New York: John Wiley & Sons.

Bower, B. (1996, July 13). Rational mind designs. *Science News, 150,* 24–25.

Breen, B. (2000a, September). (Really) risky business. *Fast Company,* 304.

Breen, B. (2000b, September). What's your intuition? *Fast Company, 290*.

British Medical Association. (1987). *Living with risk: The British Medical Association Guide*. Chichester, UK: John Wiley & Sons.

Bucher, H. C., Weinbacher, M., & Gyr, K. (1994). Influence of method of reporting study results on decision of physicians to prescribe drugs to lower cholesterol concentration. *British Medical Journal, 309*(6957), 761–764.

Cahalan, D., & Room, R. (1974). *Problem drinking among American men*. New Brunswick, NJ: Rutgers Center of Alcohol Studies.

Cleary, P. D. (1987). Why people take precautions against health risks. In N. D. Weinstein (Ed.), *Taking care: Understanding and encouraging self-protective behavior* (pp. 119–149). Cambridge, UK: Cambridge University Press.

Cohen, M. S. (1993). Three paradigms for viewing decision biases. In G. A. Klein, J. Orasanu, R. Calderwood, & C. E. Zsambok (Eds.), *Decision making in action: Models and methods* (pp. 36–50). Norwood, NJ: Ablex Publishing Corporation.

Collins, R., Peto, R., MacMahon, S., Hebert, P., Fiebach, N. H., Eberlein, K. A., et al. (1990). Blood pressure, stroke, and coronary heart disease. Part 2, Short-term reductions in blood pressure: Overview of randomised drug trials in their epidemiological context. *Lancet, 335*(8693), 827–838.

Connors, G. J., O'Farrell, T. J., Cutter, H. S., & Thompson, D. L. (1987). Dose-related effects of alcohol among male alcoholics, problem drinkers and nonproblem drinkers. *Journal of Studies on Alcohol, 48*(5), 461–466.

Critchlow, B. (1987). A utility analysis of drinking. *Addictive Behaviors, 12*(3), 269–273.

Edwards, A., Elwyn, G., Covey, J., Matthews, E., & Pill, R. (2001). Presenting risk information—A review of the effects of "framing" and other manipulations on patient outcomes. *Journal of Health Communication, 6*(1), 61–82.

Epstein, S. (1994). Integration of the cognitive and the psychodynamic unconscious. *American Psychologist, 49*(8), 709–724.

Fisher, B., Costantino, J. P., Wickerham, D. L., Redmond, C. K., Kavanah, M., Cronin, W. M., et al. (1998). Tamoxifen for prevention of breast cancer: Report of the National Surgical Adjuvant Breast and Bowel Project P-1 Study. *Journal of the National Cancer Institute, 90*(18), 1371–1388.

Gigerenzer, G. (2000). *Adaptive thinking: Rationality in the real world*. New York: Oxford University Press.

Gigerenzer, G. (2002). *Calculated risks: How to know when numbers deceive you*. New York: Simon & Schuster.

Gilovich, T., & Griffin, D. (2002). Introduction—Heuristics and biases: Then and now. In T. Gilovich, D. Griffin, & D. Kahneman (Eds.), *Heuristics and biases: The psychology of intuitive judgment* (pp. 1–18). Cambridge, UK: Cambridge University Press.

Gilovich, T., Griffin, D., & Kahneman, D. (Eds.). (2002). *Heuristics and biases: The psychology of intuitive judgment*. Cambridge, UK: Cambridge University Press.

Gonzalez, G. M., & Haney, M. L. (1990). Perceptions of risk as predictors of alcohol, marijuana, and cocaine use among college students. *Journal of College Student Development, 31,* 313–318.

Graham, J. D., & Wiener, J. B. (1995). Confronting risk tradeoffs. In J. D. Graham & J. B. Wiener (Eds.), *Risk vs. risk: Tradeoffs in protecting health and the environment* (pp. 1–41). Cambridge, MA: Harvard University Press.

Greenfield, T. K., & Rogers, J. D. (1999). Alcoholic beverage choice, risk perception and self-reported drunk driving: Effects of measurement on risk analysis. *Addiction, 94*(11), 1735–1743.

Gustafson, R. (1991). Is the strength and the desirability of alcohol-related expectancies positively related? A test with an adult Swedish sample. *Drug & Alcohol Dependence, 28*(2), 145–150.

Gustafson, R. (1993). Alcohol-related expected effects and the desirability of these effects for Swedish college students measured with the Alcohol Expectancy Questionnaire (AEQ). *Alcohol & Alcoholism, 28*(4), 469–475.

Guyatt, G., & Rennie, D. (2002). *Users' guides to the medical literature: A manual for evidence-based clinical practice.* Chicago: American Medical Association.

Hacking, I. (1975). *The emergence of probability: A philosophical study of early ideas about probability, induction, and statistical inference.* London: Cambridge University Press.

Hájek, A. (2001). Pascal's Wager. In E. Zalta (Ed.), *The Stanford Encyclopedia of Philosophy.* Retrieved August 21, 2003, from http://plato.stanford.edu/archives/win2001/entries/ pascal-wager.

Heinonen, O. P., Huttunen, J. K., Manninen, V., Manttari, M., Koskinen, P., Tenkanen, L., et al. (1994). The Helsinki Heart Study: Coronary heart disease incidence during an extended follow-up. *Journal of Internal Medicine, 235*(1), 41–49.

Hux, J. E., & Naylor, C. D. (1995). Communicating the benefits of chronic preventive therapy: Does the format of efficacy data determine patients' acceptance of treatment? *Medical Decision Making, 15*(2), 152–157.

Janz, N. K., & Becker, M. H. (1984). The Health Belief Model: A decade later. *Health Education Quarterly, 11*(1), 1–47.

Jeffery, R. W. (1989). Risk behaviors and health. Contrasting individual and population perspectives. *American Psychologist, 44*(9), 1194–1202.

Jones, B. M., & Vega, A. (1972). Cognitive performance measured on the ascending and descending limb of the blood alcohol curve. *Psychopharmacologia, 23*(2), 99–114.

Jones, B. T., & McMahon, J. (1994a). Negative alcohol expectancy predicts post-treatment abstinence survivorship: The whether, when and why of relapse to a first drink. *Addiction, 89*(12), 1653–1665.

Jones, B. T., & McMahon, J. (1994b). Negative and positive alcohol expectancies as predictors of abstinence after discharge from a residential treatment program: A one-month and three-month follow-up study in men. *Journal of Studies on Alcohol, 55*(5), 543–548.

Jones, B. T., & McMahon, J. (1996a). Changes in alcohol expectancies during treatment relate to subsequent abstinence survivorship. *British Journal of Clinical Psychology, 35*(Pt. 2), 221–234.

Jones, B. T., & McMahon, J. (1996b). A comparison of positive and negative alcohol expectancy and value and their multiplicative composite as predictors of post-treatment abstinence survivorship. *Addiction, 91*(1), 89–99.

Kahneman, D., Slovic, P., & Tversky, A. (1982). *Judgment under uncertainty: Heuristics and biases.* Cambridge, UK: Cambridge University Press.

Kahneman, D., & Tversky, A. (1984). Choices, values, and frames. *American Psychologist, 39*, 341–350.

Kahneman, D., & Tversky, A. (2000). Choices, values, and frames. In D. Kahneman & A. Tversky (Eds.), *Choices, values, and frames* (pp. 1–16). Cambridge, UK: Cambridge University Press.

Kammen, D. M., & Hassenzahl, D. M. (1999). *Should we risk it? Exploring environmental, health, and technological problem solving.* Princeton, NJ: Princeton University Press.

Keeney, R. L. (1994). Decisions about life-threatening risks. *New England Journal of Medicine, 331*(3), 193–196.

Klein, G. A. (1998). *Sources of power: How people make decisions.* Cambridge, MA: The MIT Press.

Klein, G. A., Orasanu, J., Calderwood, R., & Zsambok, C. E. (Eds.). (1993). *Decision making in action: Models and methods.* Norwood, NJ: Ablex Publishing Corporation.

Leigh, B. C. (1987). Beliefs about the effects of alcohol on self and others. *Journal of Studies on Alcohol, 48*(5), 467–475.

Leigh, B. C. (1989). Attitudes and expectancies as predictors of drinking habits: A comparison of three scales. *Journal of Studies on Alcohol, 50*(5), 432–440.

Leigh, B. C., & Stacy, A. W. (1994). Self-generated alcohol expectancies in four samples of drinkers. *Addiction Research, 1,* 335–348.

Loewenstein, G. F. (1999). A visceral account of addiction. In J. Elster & O.-J. Skog (Eds.), *Getting hooked: Rationality and addiction.* Cambridge, UK: Cambridge University Press.

Malenka, D. J., Baron, J. A., Johansen, S., Wahrenberger, J. W., & Ross, J. M. (1993). The framing effect of relative and absolute risk. *Journal of General Internal Medicine, 8*(10), 543–548.

Mann, L. M., Chassin, L., & Sher, K. J. (1987). Alcohol expectancies and the risk for alcoholism. *Journal of Consulting & Clinical Psychology, 55*(3), 411–417.

Marlatt, G. A. (1987). Alcohol, the magic elixir: Stress, expectancy, and the transformation of emotional states. In E. Gottheil, K. A. Druley, S. Pashko, & S. P. Weinstein (Eds.), *Stress and addiction* (pp. 302–322). New York: Brunner/Mazel.

Matthews, R. (1998). Hidden perils: Coping with risks to public health is fraught with danger. *New Scientist, 157*(2122), 16.

McCarty, D., Morrison, S., & Mills, K. C. (1983). Attitudes, beliefs and alcohol use: An analysis of relationships. *Journal of Studies on Alcohol, 44*(2), 328–341.

McCormack, J. P., & Levine, M. (1993). Meaningful interpretation of risk reduction from clinical drug trials. *Annals of Pharmacotherapy, 27*(10), 1272–1277.

McGettigan, P., Sly, K., O'Connell, D., Hill, S., & Henry, D. (1999). The effects of information framing on the practices of physicians. *Journal of General Internal Medicine, 14*(10), 633–642.

McMahon, J., & Jones, B. T. (1994). Negative expectancy in motivation. *Addiction Research, 1,* 145–155.

McMahon, J., & Jones, B. T. (1996). Post-treatment abstinence survivorship and motivation for recovery: The predictive validity of the Readiness to Change (RCQ) and Negative Alcohol Expectancy (NAEQ) questionnaires. *Addiction Research, 4*(2), 161–176.

McMahon, J., Jones, B. T., & O'Donnell, P. (1994). Comparing positive and negative alcohol expectancies in male and female social drinkers. *Addiction Research, 1*(4), 349–365.

McNeil, B. J., Pauker, S. G., Sox, H. C., Jr., & Tversky, A. (1982). On the elicitation of preferences for alternative therapies. *New England Journal of Medicine, 306*(21), 1259–1262.

Mello, N. K. (1968). Some aspects of the behavioral pharmacology of alcohol. In D. H. Efron (Ed.), *Psychopharmacology: A review of progress* (Public Health Service Publication No. 1863, pp. 787–809). Washington, DC: U.S. Government Printing Office.

Misselbrook, D., & Armstrong, D. (2001). Patients' responses to risk information about the benefits of treating hypertension. *British Journal of General Practice, 51*(465), 276–279.

Morris, L. A., Swasy, J. L., & Mazis, M. B. (1994). Accepted risk and alcohol use during pregnancy. *Journal of Consumer Research, 21*(1), 135–144.

National Research Council. (1996). *Understanding risk: Informing decisions in a democratic society.* Washington, DC: National Academy Press.

Nelkin, D. (1989). Communicating technological risk: The social construction of risk perception. *Annual Review of Public Health, 10,* 95–113.

Orasanu, J., & Connolly, T. (1993). The reinvention of decision making. In G. A. Klein, J. Orasanu, R. Calderwood, & C. E. Zsambok (Eds.), *Decision making in action: Models and methods* (pp. 3–20). Norwood, NJ: Ablex Publishing Corporation.

Pascal, B. (1910). *Pascal's Pensées* (W. F. Trotter, Trans.). New York: Collier. (Original work published in 1669.)

Rockhill, B. (2001). The privatization of risk. *American Journal of Public Health, 91*(3), 365–368.

Rogers, R. W. (1983). Cognitive and psychological processes in fear appeals and attitude change: A revised theory of protection motivation. In J. T. Cacioppo & R. E. Petty (Eds.), *Social psychophysiology* (pp. 153–176). New York: Guilford Press.

Roizen, R. (1983). Loosening up: General population views of the effects of alcohol. In R. Room & G. Collins (Eds.), *Alcohol and disinhibition: Nature and meaning of the link* (Vol. NIAAA, Research Monograph No. 12, pp. 236–257). Washington, DC: U.S. Government Printing Office.

Room, R., Bondy, S. J., & Ferris, J. (1995). The risk of harm to oneself from drinking, Canada 1989. *Addiction, 90,* 499–513.

Rose, G. (1981). Strategy of prevention: Lessons from cardiovascular disease. *British Medical Journal (Clinical Research Edition), 282*(6279), 1847–1851.

Rose, G. (1985). Sick individuals and sick populations. *International Journal of Epidemiology, 14*(1), 32–38.

Sackett, D. L., & Cook, R. J. (1994). Understanding clinical trials. *British Medical Journal, 309*(6957), 755–756.

Savage, L. J. (1954). *The foundations of statistics.* New York: John Wiley.

Schwarz, N. (1988). How do I feel about it? The informative function of affective states. In K. Fiedler & J. Forgas (Eds.), *Affect, cognition and social behavior: New evidence and integrative attempts* (pp. 44–62). Toronto: C. J. Hogrefe.

Schwarz, N. (2002). Feelings as information: Moods influence judgments and processing strategies. In T. Gilovich, D. Griffin, & D. Kahneman (Eds.), *Heuristics and biases: The psychology of intuitive judgment* (pp. 534–547). Cambridge, UK: Cambridge University Press.

Sedlmeier, P. (1999). *Improving statistical reasoning: Theoretical models and practical implications.* Mahwah, NJ: Lawrence Erlbaum.

Siegrist, M. (1997). Communicating low risk magnitudes: Incidence rates expressed as frequency versus rates expressed as probability. *Risk Analysis,* 17, 507–510.

Sjöberg, L. (1998). Risk perception of alcohol consumption. *Alcoholism: Clinical and Experimental Research, 22*(Suppl. 7), 277S–284S.

Skolbekken, J.-A. (1998). Communicating the risk reduction achieved by cholesterol reducing drugs. *British Medical Journal, 316*(7149), 1956–1958.

Slovic, P. (2001). Cigarette smokers: Rational actors or rational fools? In P. Slovic (Ed.), *Smoking: Risk, perception, and policy* (pp. 97–124). Thousand Oaks, CA: Sage Publications.

Slovic, P., Finucane, M., Peters, E., & MacGregor, D. G. (2002). The affect heuristic. In T. Gilovich, D. Griffin, & D. Kahneman (Eds.), *Heuristics and biases: The psychology of intuitive judgment* (pp. 397–420). Cambridge, UK: Cambridge University Press.

Slovic, P., Finucane, M., Peters, E., & MacGregor, D. (2004). Risk as analysis and risk as feelings: Some thoughts about affect, reason, risk, and rationality. *Risk Analysis.*

Slovic, P., Fischhoff, B., & Lichtenstein, S. (1978). Accident probabilities and seat belt usage: A psychological perspective. *Accident Analysis and Prevention, 10,* 281–285.

Slovic, P., Fischhoff, B., & Lichtenstein, S. (2000a). Cognitive processes and societal risk taking. In P. Slovic (Ed.), *The perception of risk* (pp. 32–50). London: Earthscan Publications.

Slovic, P., Fischhoff, B., & Lichtenstein, S. (2000b). Response mode, framing and information-processing effects in risk assessment. In P. Slovic (Ed.), *The perception of risk* (pp. 154–167). London: Earthscan Publications.

Slovic, P., Kunreither, H., & White, G. F. (2000). Decision processes, rationality and adjustment to natural hazards. In P. Slovic (Ed.), *The perception of risk* (pp. 1–31). London: Earthscan Publications.

Stacy, A. W. (1986). *Attitude and expectancy models of alcohol use: An integration of theoretical perspectives.* Unpublished doctoral dissertation, University of California, Riverside, CA.

Stacy, A. W., & Widaman, K. F. (1987). A "positivity" bias in attitude models of alcohol use. *Annual Meeting of the American Psychological Association,* New York.

Stacy, A. W., Widaman, K. F., & Marlatt, G. A. (1990). Expectancy models of alcohol use. *Journal of Personality & Social Psychology, 58*(5), 918–928.

Steiner, J. F. (1999). Talking about treatment: The language of populations and the language of individuals. *Annals of Internal Medicine, 130*(7), 618–622.

Stutts, M. A., Patterson, L. T., & Hunnicutt, G. G. (1997). Females' perception of risks associated with alcohol consumption during pregnancy. *American Journal of Health Behavior, 21*(2), 137–146.

Testa, M., & Reifman, A. (1996). Individual differences in perceived riskiness of drinking in pregnancy: Antecedents and consequences. *Journal of Studies on Alcohol, 57*(4), 360–367.

Tolley, G., Kenkel, D., & Fabian, R. (Eds.). (1994). *Valuing health for policy: An economic approach.* London: University of Chicago Press.

Tversky, A., & Kahneman, D. (1974). Judgment under uncertainty: Heuristics and biases. *Science, 185,* 1124–1131.

Tversky, A., & Kahneman, D. (2000). Rational choice and the framing of decisions. In D. Kahneman & A. Tversky (Eds.), *Choices, values, and frames* (pp. 209–223). Cambridge, UK: Cambridge University Press.

Weinstein, N. D. (1987). Cross-hazard consistencies: Conclusions about self-protective behavior. In N. D. Weinstein (Ed.), *Taking care: Understanding and encouraging self-protective behavior* (pp. 325–335). Cambridge, UK: Cambridge University Press.

Weinstein, N. D. (1989). Perceptions of personal susceptibility to harm. In V. M. Mays, G. W. Albee, & S. F. Schneider (Eds.), *Primary prevention of AIDS* (pp. 142–167). Newbury Park, CA: Sage.

Weinstein, N. D. (1993). Testing four competing theories of health-protective behavior. *Health Psychology, 12*(4), 324–333.

Weinstein, N. D., & Nicolich, M. (1993). Correct and incorrect interpretations of correlations between risk perceptions and risk behaviors. *Health Psychology, 12*(3), 235–245.

Wieczorek, W. F., Mirand, A. L., & Callahan, C. P. (1994). Perception of the risk of arrest for drinking and driving. *Criminal Justice and Behavior, 21*(3), 312–324.

Wild, T. C., & Cunningham, J. (2001). Psychosocial determinants of perceived vulnerability to harm among adult drinkers. *Journal of Studies on Alcohol, 62*(1), 105–113.

Wild, T. C., Hinson, R., Cunningham, J., & Bacchiochi, J. (2001). Perceived vulnerability to alcohol-related harm in young adults: Independent effects of risky alcohol use and drinking motives. *Experimental and Clinical Psychopharmacology, 9*(1), 117–125.

Young, R. M., & Knight, R. G. (1989). The Drinking Expectancy Questionnaire: A revised measure of alcohol-related beliefs. *Journal of Psychopathology & Behavioral Assessment, 11*(1), 99–112.

Zajonc, R. B. (1980). Feeling and thinking: Preferences need no inferences. *American Psychologist, 35,* 151–175.

Chapter 6

Toeing the Line: Risk and Alcohol Policy

When individuals are confronted with risk, they respond by assessing potential harms, weighing these against potential benefits, and making a decision based on the balance. For each of us, this balance is different, and it is colored by many of the factors discussed in the earlier chapters of this book. When it comes to societal risks, however, the equation becomes more complex. Societies must balance the competing concerns of individuals, determine which risks and which responses are feasible, and make judgments on where the threshold between acceptable and unacceptable risk lies.

Many of the risks we now recognize as being the concern of society as a whole were once considered part of exclusive domain of individual responsibility. Riding in automobiles without seat belts, engaging in unprotected sex, and smoking around those who do not are today recognized as having consequences that extend well beyond those persons who are immediately involved. The evolution of definitions of risk and responsibility has given rise to concepts such as "social cost," which are closely linked with decisions about policy approaches to manage the risks facing society.

Policy measures relating to risk have been implemented in a wide range of areas that affect the daily lives of individuals. They extend from food safety and health issues to social welfare, the design of vehicles, development of infrastructure, political balance, and environmental issues. Such policies aim to establish a framework within which risks can be addressed and delineate roles for the players involved in executing the policies. Policies must take into account risk assessment, risk management, and risk communication. If policies are to be effective, however, they must also factor in the gut response of individuals to risks and consider the public's response to any implemented measures as well as the palatability of particular approaches to risk management.

In this regard, alcohol policies are no different from any other policies. Public and private pressures, as well as individual and societal concerns, come into play in the development of policy approaches aimed at risks associated with certain patterns of drinking. This chapter attempts to position alcohol policy within the broader context of public policy approaches relating to risk and to examine their theoretical underpinnings.

WHO ARE THE PLAYERS? SOCIAL RESPONSIBILITY AND A RESPONSIBLE SOCIETY

The debate surrounding policy approaches to risk management reflects prevailing views on who bears the ultimate responsibility for preserving the well-being of both society and the individual. Thus, before beginning any discussion on how risk management policies, particularly those associated with alcohol consumption, are designed and implemented, it is necessary to first examine the key players and their respective roles in the process of policy development.

At opposing ends of the spectrum lie two views on the nature of the relationship between risk and public policy. The politically "liberal" view contends that the burden of responsibility lies with society as a whole. This applies not only to responsibility for managing risks, but also for preventing them in the first place. The politically "conservative" position is generally associated with a greater emphasis on individual freedoms, along with individual responsibility for managing risk and harm. In reality, most policies lie somewhere between these two extremes.

The traditional view of risk management and policy response development in many parts of the world is based largely on the notion of collective sharing of rights and responsibilities. As a result, emphasis is placed on a state-centered response to meeting risks, for both society and the individual. In recent years, however, a gradual shift away from a heavy reliance on government to an increased commitment and involvement by a range of entities has occurred—notably, the private sector, the nongovernmental sector, and individuals themselves. The degree to which these various groups are included in the process of decision making involving risk depends on broader philosophical notions about the relationship between the public and private spheres and between individuals and societal entities. Ultimately, these views also inform as well as drive the policy approaches that are adopted in managing risks.

According to social theorists, societal responsibility, especially in the face of risk, has undergone a shift that largely stems from globalization and accompanying economic, political, and cultural changes. Individual governments are no longer as free as they once were to pursue their own independent social and economic policies. As discussed in Chapter 4, the public is increasingly wary of government institutions and the individuals entrusted with the welfare of citizens (Edwards & Glover, 2001; Franklin, 1998).

Another factor that has influenced this shift is the dramatic growth in the accessibility and distribution of information. Scientific, social, and political debates have increasingly moved into the public domain, largely by design. The figurative shrinking of our world through information allows and, at the same time, forces us to view risks on a global level, as well as locally and individually. It also represents a potent driving force behind the development of policies designed to address risk and requires flexibility in the approaches that are chosen to manage them. Finally, and perhaps most important, the notion of accountability now transcends traditional boundaries and has moved into the realm of societal institutions. Governments, as well as the private sector, are increasingly held accountable for their actions and charged with the responsibility of managing risk.

National Governments

Clearly, government is a key player in managing and communicating risk (see Chapter 4). One of the principal roles of government is to ensure the safety of its citizens and to protect them from outside forces and threats. This applies equally to government's role in safeguarding the stability of financial institutions, protecting the population from military aggression or acts of terrorism, and ensuring that the day-to-day safety and well-being of individuals are met through product and workplace safety.

The role of government in public risk management, on the one hand, consists of reducing the actual risks to which people are exposed and, on the other, reallocating risks away from those who are most vulnerable to them. Prohibiting or controlling certain activities most often achieves risk reduction. Safety regulations governing the disposal of hazardous or radioactive materials are an example of government supervision that extends into everyday life, as are standards for cleanliness and food preparation in restaurants or guidelines for health workers with regard to the patients in their care.

Other strategies rely on reallocating risk away from vulnerable groups by attempting to shift exposure away from them or to spread the risk across a larger segment of the population. This second approach underlies measures such as social insurance or liability. In some cases, risk reallocation can also be an effective means of risk reduction (Moss, 2002). Risk management often involves a balance between these two approaches. The direction in which the scale is tipped and the extent to which government plays a role in the equation vary from country to country.

Governments differ in how they respond to risk, mirroring the prevailing notions among their constituencies about the degree of government involvement that is acceptable. In Sweden, for example, policies aimed at managing risk can be implemented in a largely proactive way (Sjöberg, 1998). A high level of government control designed to manage risks and minimize harm is acceptable to the public. In the U.S., however, an approach that relies heavily on government involvement is generally not palatable. As a result, government tends to be largely reactive, with action occurring only when sufficient political pressure has surrounded a particular issue or risk (Shubik, 1991, cited in Sjöberg, 1998).

Regardless of where a particular government might lie on the spectrum from paternalism to laissez-faire, it still has a significant role to play in managing risk, which it may exercise to a greater or lesser extent. Governments have an important mandate to help individuals make informed choices about potential risks, both to themselves and to others. Governments are also responsible for protecting those who are vulnerable or unable to make their own choices or decisions. Foremost among these groups are children and young people, or those whose physical or emotional state does not allow them to make their own decisions about risk. Others include socially excluded groups, such as indigenous populations in many countries, who may be particularly at risk. The provision of care for those who have suffered harm may also fall within the responsibility of government, although the extent to which this is acceptable may vary. Finally, government has an important place when it comes to striking a balance between respecting individual choice and protecting society from harm and avoidable costs.

Intergovernmental Organizations

It must be recognized that government involvement in risk management can only be effective up to a certain point, especially in an age in which the fates of nations are so closely intertwined. Beyond that point, other useful approaches rely on the involvement of other, often nontraditional, players. It has become increasingly clear and more generally accepted that effective alcohol policies must also include broader and more global concerns. As a result, the role of intergovernmental institutions and their related bodies in proposing or setting policy around risk has grown significantly. These organizations now set the tone for much of what is implemented at the national level—be it to restrain the spread of HIV/AIDS, reduce the risk from land mines, or address the threat of global terrorism.

The mounting involvement of global players has been, in large part, driven by the expansion of trade and the exchange of information, as well as by increasingly overlapping political interests. Policy development now transcends the physical boundaries of individual countries. To an expanding degree, policy at the national level is predicated upon or influenced by approaches developed at the regional or global level, with local interests often deferring to global ones. This trend toward global (or macro) approaches is witnessed by the increasing involvement of intergovernmental organizations in the development of policy that focuses on alcohol and other issues affecting society.

The World Trade Organization (WTO) is actively involved in issues of global trade and the free market, as well as commercial aspects of policy development. Trade agreements, once the domain of individual states, are now the bailiwick of the General Agreements on Tariffs and Trade (GATT) and the General Agreements on Trade in Services (GATS). Yet, global involvement comes at a price, as global approaches go head to head with those traditionally implemented by sovereign states.

One such example is offered by the state-run monopolies that control alcohol sales in a handful of European countries (i.e., Sweden, Iceland, Finland, and the Faroe Islands), as well as in some jurisdictions of the U.S. and Canada. Within the globalized world of alcohol policy, the existence of monopolies is at odds with the notion of free enterprise, creating some conflict, such as in the efforts to harmonize policies across member states of the European Union (EU). The ensuing tension between those who favor relaxing regulation and the proponents of traditional entities and approaches is significantly changing the landscape for policy development (Österberg & Karlsson, 2002; Room, 2001; *Sweden v. European Commission*, 2000).

Public health and social policy within the alcohol field also creates divided loyalties between the national-level priorities of governments and their concerns and agendas on a global scale. For example, the World Health Organization (WHO) Regional Office for Europe, closely involved in the development and implementation of alcohol policies to address health issues and reduce social cost, launched the European Alcohol Action Plan (EAAP) in 1992 (World Health Organization [WHO], 1993). This document marked the beginning of a coordinated policy approach at the international level. There has since been an effort to implement the elements outlined in this plan—health promotion, primary health care, and public policies on alcohol—at the country level. In 1995, member states in the European region adopted the European Charter on Alcohol (WHO, 1995), outlining several national strategies for controlling potential problems, all based on similar principles. To date, no equivalent initiative exists in any other region of the world.

Although they stem from common commercial, political, and health concerns, such policy approaches are also a double-edged sword. On the one hand, it can be argued that a global approach may be more effective than individual country initiatives. On the other, the involvement of global entities, at times, may undermine the autonomy of individual states. In addition, as preceding chapters have shown, when it comes to risk, perceptions and definitions are largely culture-specific. It is therefore necessary to appreciate that approaches to the management of risk and the minimization of harm should also be culture-specific. What may be an effective policy in Norway may not be compatible with the culture in Chile; the risk priorities that need to be addressed in Zambia are quite distinct from those in New Zealand. Even in countries within the same general geographic region and with similar cultures, differences in infra-structure, socioeconomic disparities, the priority given alcohol problems on the scale of relevant risks, and resources available to implement change may be widely divergent.

The Private Sector

During his address to the World Economic Forum in Davos, Switzerland, in January 1998, United Nations Secretary-General Kofi Annan challenged world business leaders to help build the social and environmental pillars required to sustain the new global economy and make globalization work for all the world's people:

> Leaders of government and business continue to have choices. So let us choose to unite the power of markets with the authority of universal ideas. Let us choose to reconcile the creative forces of private entrepreneurship with the needs of the disadvantaged and the requirements of future generations. Let us ensure that prosperity reaches the poor. Let us choose an enlightened way forward towards our ultimate, shared goal: a global market place that is open to all and benefits all.

This call to action by the U.N. Secretary-General highlights a shift that has been occurring gradually in an effort to broaden responsibility for the well-being of society beyond governments and other public institutions. Formerly nontraditional partners now have an increasing joint role to play in addressing and reducing potential risks. Corporations and the private sector, in general, are becoming very much a part of the equation, particularly when it comes to safeguarding against potential risks inherent in technology, industrialization, and individual products. There exists a strong view that corporations have some measure of responsibility, be it moral or legal, to address both the beneficial and deleterious effects their products may have on society. Industrialized societies within the developed world expect and demand that corporations meet certain standards. At the same time, a clear recognition also exists within these corporations that social responsibility and good corporate citizenship constitute good business practice.

The responsibility of the private sector in the face of risk can either be imposed by legislation and enforcement through government oversight or it can be self-directed. Numerous self-regulatory codes and standards exist as an incentive for industries to hold themselves responsible for their own conduct, for the consumer products and durable goods they produce, and for the services they offer. Notably, the investment sector in the U.S. has successfully regulated its own practices concerning the trading of securities and commodities through entities such as the New York Stock Exchange (NYSE) and the National Association of Securities Dealers (NASD).

Similarly, the Motion Picture Association of America has implemented a voluntary ratings system for films that speaks to their appropriateness for young audiences.

Self-regulation can be as useful a tool for the beverage alcohol industry as it is in others.. The industry has made numerous efforts to establish an effective mechanism for self-regulation, both industry-wide and within individual companies. To date, self-regulation in the alcohol field has been largely confined to advertising and marketing practices. The challenge is to adapt self-regulatory approaches to the conditions prevailing in different markets, either mature or emerging, and to ensure that common standards are upheld equally in all of them (International Center for Alcohol Policies [ICAP], 2001, 2002). Like many other commodities, beverage alcohol, when misused, can carry considerable potential for harm. As a result, it is in the beverage alcohol industry's best interest to ensure that these risks are managed and that the potential for harm is minimized. In addition, for the alcohol industry, as well as for any other entity within the private sector, self-regulation is preferable to government regulation; however, it should be recognized that when self-regulatory efforts fail, government intervention might be an appropriate response.

Successful self-regulation relies on both a comprehensive code of conduct and an independent mechanism for monitoring and enforcing compliance. An effective approach has been implemented by The Portman Group, a beverage alcohol industry-sponsored organization in the United Kingdom that monitors the marketing practices of its member companies and responds to complaints lodged by the public, especially when it comes to the marketing of novelty products. The Portman Group's Code of Practice on the Naming, Packaging and Promotion of Alcoholic Drinks (The Portman Group, 2003b) was introduced in April 1996 and revised several times over the intervening years in an attempt to ensure the responsible marketing of beverage alcohol. To date, more than 130 beverage producers and retailers have signed up to register their support for the Code. Any complaints lodged are considered by the Independent Complaints Panel and published in an Annual Code Report. As a means of enforcement, retailers are requested to cease stocking the offending products, thus pressuring producers into compliance.

It is important, however, to note that self-regulation and government regulation are not mutually exclusive. The effectiveness of both approaches in minimizing risk relies on finding the right balance between government regulation and industry's acknowledgment that it is accountable for its own actions. Industry self-policing and government regulation need to coexist on a continuum. How far the scale is tipped in favor of one over the other depends on the effectiveness of the self-regulatory process, the political climate, the culture involved, and prevailing views within a particular society.

A Role for the Public

Most traditional policy approaches to risk management are implemented in a "top-down" fashion. Generally developed by government, they are directed at the public, creating a one-way flow from "experts" at the top of the hierarchy and the "lay public" at the bottom. Yet, the public's gut reaction to risk is a powerful force—one not to be discounted. People need a voice in the things that matter to them, that cause them fear and concern, and that relate directly to their lives. Effective policy measures, therefore, need to be designed with possible public reaction in mind. In order to be useful, policy needs to make sense. Although the design of alcohol policies certainly needs to reflect the involvement of national governments and global organizations, as well as private and nongovernmental sectors, at the end of the day, the ultimate decision of whether or not to drink rests with the individual.

To have the desired impact, policy approaches need to correspond to the actual experience of individuals and be relevant within the context of their lives. With regard to alcohol, this means policies should factor in the role of alcohol within a particular society, and be compatible with how people actually drink and the risks they perceive in relation to alcohol. Individuals should have a choice in making the ultimate decisions about their own drinking, provided these decisions do not infringe upon the choices or safety of those around them. "Choice (also known as decision making) is the essence of intelligent, purposeful behavior" (Slovic, 1990). With the introduction of choice, managing risk becomes a moral enterprise.

The main role of society and its institutions, then, is to equip individuals with the tools necessary to make informed and responsible decisions. These tools should include full and balanced information about alcohol and the potential consequences of drinking. At the same time, it is also up to society to ensure that the choices of the few do not interfere with the freedom and the safety of the many.

Other Players

Other players also have a key role in developing policies designed to manage and minimize risk. In the alcohol field, as in any health-related area, researchers, health, and medical professionals are needed to make informed policy decisions about risk and to implement many of those measures. Their essential roles in risk communication were already discussed in Chapter 4.

Advocacy groups, religious organizations, consumer groups, and civil society organizations also play a vital role in shaping alcohol policy. Yet, philosophical issues may complicate the involvement of such groups because many such entities represent particular ideological positions, particularly when it comes to alcohol. As a result, the legitimacy of their involvement in

the shaping of policy is being debated, although such groups wield considerable influence and can be highly effective.

POLICY APPROACHES TO RISK

The so-called Precautionary Principle has shaped much of the current
thinking on policies that involve risk management. Based on the German
Vorsorgeprinzip (literally, "foresight planning principle"), this concept was
first developed in the 1970s within the context of environmental policy
(de Sadeleer, 2002). According to the *Vorsorgeprinzip*, a distinction exists
between human actions that cause "dangers" and those that cause "risks."
Dangers are to be prevented at all costs, while risks require detailed analysis
to determine whether preventative action is appropriate. In its original form,
the principle was applied to governmental oversight and action, particularly
in areas in which the public was considered inadequately prepared or unable
to make certain decisions (Aichmayer & Schindler, 2002). It has become increasingly relevant, however, to the actions of the private sector as an
approach to risk management within the realms of public health and environmental policy.

At what point the Precautionary Principle should be applied has generated some disagreement. One view is that action should be taken *despite*
scientific uncertainty, avoiding a so-called "paralysis of analysis" where
insufficient evidence or understanding of risks is an excuse for inaction
(Aichmayer & Schindler, 2002). The other view regarding the implementation of the Precautionary Principle considers it an appropriate measure only
when there is a sufficient body of credible evidence that serious or irreversible damage to health or the environment could be caused. This position
holds that sound scientific principles and a thorough cost–benefit analysis
need to inform what levels of risk are acceptable and what action needs to be
taken. Industry and government should share any decisions. The final deter-
mination should not be contingent on the need to prove an absence of risk,
and should be carried out within a legal framework that ensures transparency. Any measures taken in this approach should be proportional to the
degree of potential risk. Restrictive measures are a last resort only after less
restrictive ones have proven inadequate.

Clearly, the Precautionary Principle spans a broad range of positions
from the "strong" approach, according to which risks should never be
taken, to the "weak" approach, primarily an injunction to be prudent and
err on the side of caution when it comes to taking risks (Morris, 2000). As a
result, the Precautionary Principle has been criticized for politicizing
science and for being applied in cases in which the science is "uncertain"
and the available evidence "insufficient" (European Policy Center, 1999).
Although the Precautionary Principle has generally been implemented in
areas such as food technology (e.g., in the debate over genetically modified

organisms) and the nuclear industry, its underlying principles are also reflected in many alcohol policy approaches aimed at preventing harm and diminishing risks.

Controversy surrounds the relationship between the Precautionary Principle and the development of policy. To some, it represents an excuse for government and other entities to curtail the freedom of the individual and restrain free enterprise. Others believe the Precautionary Principle can be used to increase safety and reduce risks, that it strengthens the credibility of science as a tool for risk assessment and management, and ensures the legitimacy, predictability, and transparency of the regulatory process. Finally, for some, the Precautionary Principle is an example of a modern paradox that although most of us may be safer today than ever before, we spend more time worrying about our safety.

Risk Management through Alcohol Policy

In practice, policies aimed at managing risk, including those relating to alcohol consumption, can be divided into two basic categories. The first is a top-down approach relying heavily on government and its institutions with an emphasis on legislation, controls, enforcement, and punitive measures. It stems from a general position that responsibility for risk management is shared and should be addressed through government. Inherent in this model is the dichotomy between the "experts" who make policy decisions and the "lay public," to whom decisions about risks and their management are handed down.

The second approach makes use of a broader and more inclusive base of players, involving communities and the public. It emphasizes education and measures that are intended to change behavior in an effort to manage risk. Central to this approach is the way it addresses concerns that are relevant to the public. Decisions about risk are not left in the hands of "experts" alone; instead, the public is allowed to make many of its own decisions about risk and assume some of the responsibility. In addition, entities such as non-governmental organizations and the private sector are also included in the process. It should be noted, however, that despite the different emphasis and strategies employed in these two approaches, they are not mutually exclusive. Each has its own strengths and weaknesses, and neither is effective in isolation from the other. Integration of the two approaches is possible, and, in practice, exists to some degree in most comprehensive policy models.

Alcohol Control Policies

Most traditional approaches to alcohol policy rely heavily on a top-down approach in their formulation. In this sense, they do not differ vastly from policy approaches that have been implemented in a number of other fields. Government is viewed as primarily responsible for the decisions that are

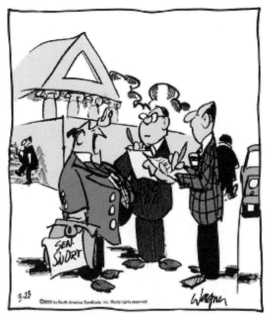

"How we conduct the people's business is none of the people's business!"

aimed at controlling risk and protecting the population. Limiting the availability of alcohol is viewed as a means of reducing the incidence of problems and the risk for harm. The approach relies on government intervention through legislation and punitive measures. Based on the "control of consumption" or "single-distribution" theory, control policies are predicated upon the existence of a mathematical relationship between alcohol consumption and risk for related problems (Ledermann, 1952; Ledermann & Tabah, 1951). According to this paradigm, a fixed and predictable relationship exists between the level of average per capita alcohol consumption across a population and the incidence of problems (i.e., social or medical) within that population. The theory suggests that reducing the level of per capita consumption across groups, such as within individual countries, will lead to a reduction in the incidence of problems (Edwards et al., 1994; Saunders & de Burgh, 1998).

The simplicity of this approach to policy holds a certain appeal, and it has been extensively translated into a range of real-world measures. Because it relies on aggregate consumption representing averages across an entire population, the approach neither allows for differentiation among individuals, nor makes separate provisions for those whose drinking is associated with risk for harm and those whose drinking is not. It is a one-size-fits-all policy model, relying on blanket solutions to address specific problems that may be associated with particular groups and special subpopulations.

Control policies are implemented in a number of ways and are usually combined into a comprehensive approach that simultaneously regulates many aspects of the alcohol market. These policies are targeted at one or any combination of the following: the product itself, those who sell or provide the product, the conditions under which the product is sold or provided, and consumers of the product.

One of the most commonly used measures is to increase the price of beverage alcohol in order to drive down consumption. This is often achieved through sales and excise taxes. Reviews of the effectiveness of pricing as a means of reducing demand are mixed. Strong evidence exists that their impact may be limited only to certain subgroups of consumers. Heavy drinkers, a high-risk population, are likely to continue in their consumption patterns regardless of price, although they may shift what they consume to less expensive beverages (Manning, Blumberg, & Moulton, 1995). Similarly, those who occasionally drink very small amounts of alcohol or abstain altogether are not likely to be affected by price increases. The impact of this measure, therefore, will be felt most strongly by moderate consumers—those generally not at high risk for alcohol problems but who are more sensitive to price fluctuations.

Evidence also suggests that increasing taxes and duties on beverage alcohol also has an impact on cross-border trade. Where prices (and taxes) are high, consumers may choose to bring beverage alcohol across the border from jurisdictions where they are lower. For example, high beverage alcohol prices in Sweden are an incentive for Swedish consumers to purchase beverage alcohol from neighboring countries where prices are considerably lower. Such cross-border trade flourishes between Denmark and Sweden, aided by the recently relaxed import regulations in Sweden (Lyall, 2003). Similarly, ferries between Finland and Sweden make a detour to Finland's autonomous Aaland Islands, which are exempt from EU customs regulations and allow customers to purchase duty-free alcohol (Australian Broadcasting Corporation, 2003; European Commission, 1999). Similarly, the cross-border trade of certain types of beverage alcohol between England and France has increased dramatically as British consumers purchase less expensive products and bring them across the Channel.

High taxes and beverage alcohol prices often have consequences that are more dramatic. In areas where pricing and taxation are high, this measure may encourage illicit trade and give rise to organized crime (Haworth & Simpson, 2004). In several of the transition countries of Eastern Europe and the former Soviet republics, trade in smuggled products from cheaper markets has flourished. In addition, the manufacture of counterfeit products sold on the black market or substituted for legal commercially produced alcohol is widespread. The risk to public health because of these activities is high. In early 2002, 3 million bottles of counterfeit vodka, which were laced with methanol and packaged as legitimate imported brands, were discovered in Poland. These "pirated" bottles were available commercially for purchase by the public before they were discovered and removed (The Warsaw Voice, 2002).

In addition to pricing, several other policy measures are also aimed at reducing alcohol access and availability, including limiting the sale of alcohol through curtailed licensing hours or even banning its sale on certain days of the week or on holidays. In relation to a range of products, many governments throughout history have implemented sumptuary laws, which regulate citizens' consumption of goods for religious, moral, ethical, or economic reasons. With regard to alcohol, these laws still exist in a number of places, including the "Blue Laws" in parts of the U.S. that forbid the sale of alcohol on Sundays and holidays. These laws have their specific origin in the "Sabbatarian" laws carried on through the Puritan tradition of New England. Such rigid measures were once implemented in an effort to preserve public morality by preventing the breaking of the Sabbath, breaches in family discipline, drunkenness, and excesses in dress. Although their original intent has been lost, such laws persist and regulate the availability of beverage alcohol (Kingsley, 1871).

The U.S. is not the only country in which such measures are implemented. In Sweden, alcohol outlets were closed on Saturdays and Sundays until February 2000 in an effort to reduce sales, consumption, and problems. With EU harmonization looming, an experimental situation was created in which the impact of liberalizing restrictions on hours of sale was assessed. Over the course of 17 months, stores in certain counties were allowed to open on Saturdays. When the outcome of such liberalization was examined, a notable increase in alcohol sales occurred. Although consumption increased, however, indicators of harm directly related to alcohol consumption did not (Norström & Skog, 2003).

Other measures restricting alcohol availability are also common, including regulating the number of bars or shops that sell or serve alcohol. By limiting the number of licensed premises within a certain area, an effort is made to minimize outcomes such as drinking and driving, and violence or public disturbance (Gorman, Speer, Gruenewald, & Labouvie, 2001; Gruenewald, Johnson, & Treno, 2002; Stockwell & Gruenewald, 2001).

A number of jurisdictions in Nordic countries and North America rely on the previously mentioned state-run retail monopolies that control the distribution and pricing of alcohol. Proponents of this measure argue that monopolies allow better and more efficient control of alcohol supply and, at the same time, channel the proceeds generated through taxes and sales directly into government coffers (Byrne, 2002; Joensen, 2002; Romanus, 2002). In addition, "a government retail monopoly . . . occupies a field which otherwise would be occupied by private interests in competition with each other. The key to a monopoly's effectiveness as an instrument of the government's public order and public health aims, then, is the ways in which the monopoly's occupation of the field holds down the rates of alcohol-related problems" (Room, 2001).

An argument against the existence of alcohol monopolies focuses on issues of free enterprise and fair competition, while other criticism has been directed at the state's direct involvement in the sale of alcohol. By profiting from taxation and sales, the impartiality of the state may be compromised because high sales of beverage alcohol and the profits derived from them are in its interest. Economic motivation may appear to be at odds with the public health function of government and its role in managing risk.

Several measures exist that are directed at those who consume alcohol, instead of at the availability of the product itself. Some of these measures rely on legislation and enforcement, while others involve the criminalization of drinking and alcohol abuse. Alcohol detoxification centers providing short-term intervention for alcohol abusers exist in most countries, with varying involvement of medical assistance, treatment, and follow-up. Some of these centers are operated in conjunction with hospitals, others with police and government institutions; still others are privately funded. In many cases, admission to these centers occurs in conjunction with criminal proceedings, and it is used as a punitive measure. The approach does not offer a long-term solution for alcohol-dependent individuals in the form of intervention or treatment. Many patients in these facilities are already marginalized and socially isolated individuals for whom the often-unsafe environment in the detoxification centers creates additional problems instead of solving the basic one (Beane & Beck, 1991; Gordon et al., 2001; Rabinowitz & Marjefsky, 1998).

Measures targeted at consumers of beverage alcohol include the implementation of a minimum purchase age that restricts the sale of alcohol to those younger than this legal limit. This approach covers both drinking and purchase age, although some countries mandate these differently. Perhaps more than with most other measures, culture, the role of alcohol in society, and its general acceptability are key determinants of how drinking age is mandated. Cultural diversity explains, at least in part, why a broad range of minimum drinking ages exists around the world, from 16 years in countries such as Austria and Spain to 21 in the U.S. and Egypt (ICAP, 1998).

The effectiveness of highly restrictive purchase age limits has been criticized. Where the threshold for the allowable drinking age is held to a higher standard than the age of majority, there is an apparent disconnect in policy measures and the reasoning behind them. Whereas other behaviors, including marriage, driving, gun ownership, military service, or holding public office may be permitted at age 18, or earlier, drinking is not. In the U.S., where the legal drinking age is 21, the argument has been made that young people do not have the opportunity to learn about responsible drinking or how to integrate moderation into a healthy, normal lifestyle (Plant, 2001). An unrealistically high drinking age may be blamed, in part, for various risks to young people, such as excessive drinking or drunk driving. For example, in areas of the U.S. bordering Mexico, where the drinking age is 18, cross-border traffic to Mexican bars is high. According to some estimates (Baker, Johnson, Voas, & Lange, 2000; Voas, Lange, & Johnson, 2002), thousands of youths cross the border each night in search of legally obtainable alcohol. What this also means, however, is that cross-border traffic returning to the U.S. includes high numbers of drunk drivers and traffic accidents.

Complete prohibition of alcohol sale and consumption lie at the extreme end of alcohol control policies. Prohibition has been implemented in a number of different circumstances and for a variety of reasons. In some instances, such as in many Islamic countries, a ban on the sale of alcohol complies with religious restrictions against its consumption. In others, prohibition is used as a tool for risk management. The most notable historical example is Prohibition in the U.S., which lasted from 1920 until it was repealed in 1933. This now infamous era in American history gave rise to organized crime, and it is generally considered a failed attempt at policy. Prohibition persists in some "dry" jurisdictions, sometimes for religious or moral reasons, sometimes as vestiges of nationwide measures. In some of these areas, beverage alcohol may not be purchased but may be brought in for personal consumption, including into restaurants. In others, alcohol can neither be purchased nor consumed. An undesired side effect of this measure has been an increase, instead of a reduction, in certain types of risk. Those who wish to drink must drive to "wet" jurisdictions in order do so, increasing the likelihood of traffic accidents and drunk-driving fatalities as they return to "dry" areas. As in the previously mentioned case of cross-border traffic to and from Mexico, the relatively high frequency with which accidents occur at borders between these jurisdictions has led to the coining of the term "blood border." This border demarcates the line between areas in which alcohol is available and those in which it is restricted (Center for Substance Abuse Prevention/International Center for Alcohol Policies, 1998; Sines & Ekman, 1996).

A number of other measures are aimed at the actual product. These include requirements regarding the integrity of beverage alcohol itself and the raw materials used to produce it. These regulations are largely implemented through the manufacturers of the beverages. Although commercial beverage alcohol is generally subject to standards of purity and integrity, with brand names guaranteeing that these have been upheld, some home-produced beverages, adulteration of authentic products, and the production of illicit and counterfeit products have caused concern (Haworth & Simpson, 2004).

Finally, restrictions and bans on alcohol advertising are used not to limit supply, but to curtail demand. This approach rests on the premise that alcohol advertising encourages and increases alcohol consumption and, consequently, the risk for harm (Edwards et al., 1994). Studies from a number of countries, however, have failed to show conclusively a positive relationship between advertising and aggregate consumption of alcohol (Duffy, 1991, 1995; Fisher,

1993; Fisher & Cook, 1995; Goel & Morey, 1995; Nelson & Moran, 1995; Smith, 1990). Nevertheless, a demonstrable positive relationship exists between advertising and market share because of brand substitution (Nelson, 1997).

Because of their restrictive nature, control measures rely strongly on continuous and rigorous enforcement to be effective. Their palatability to the public reflects prevailing views on the relationship between the state and its citizens and the willingness of individuals to accept top-down approaches in which they have little involvement. Such measures prove most palatable where it is believed that governmental decisions about the good of society take precedence over the freedoms of individuals.

Drinking Patterns and Harm Reduction

It has been argued that policy approaches aimed at the general population and relying on aggregate-level measures of consumption are grossly inadequate in addressing actual risks and reducing harm (Single & Leino, 1998; Saunders & de Burgh 1998). Measures aimed at population-wide drinking levels cannot predict the relationship between the drinking patterns of specific groups of individuals and the problems that they are likely to experience. Drinking, like all things human, is shaped by many factors that also play a role in determining who is at risk and why. Cultures differ considerably with respect to both prevailing attitudes on alcohol and perceptions of risk and harm. Individuals have widely differing views on where their risk priorities lie and what measures they are willing to accept in order to make their lives potentially safer.

In recent years, a shift in focus has occurred from aggregate-level information about the drinking behavior of an entire population to the myriad drinking patterns that describe how individuals actually drink (Grant & Litvak, 1998; Single & Leino, 1998; World Health Organization [WHO], 2003). Solid evidence suggests that "patterns of drinking may be more important than levels of alcohol consumption in predicting whether people will experience problems with their drinking" (Single & Leino, 1998). Thus, the often highly individual nature of risk, especially when it comes to behaviors like alcohol consumption, can be viewed in a way that allows risk to be addressed in an individualized manner and approaches to be tailored to particular needs (Gruenewald et al., 2002; Wells & Graham, 2003).

Drinking patterns describe not just *how much* people drink, but also *how* they drink. This includes a number of variables:

• When they drink;
• Where they drink, and with whom;
• What other activities accompany their drinking (Are they drinking with a meal? Are they drinking and driving?);
• Their general health;
• Possible genetic factors that might increase certain risks;

- The effect of medications;
- Their age and gender;
- Their relative experience with drinking;
- What they are drinking—whether it is of high quality or possibly contaminated and toxic (Haworth & Simpson, 2004; Heath, 2002; Single and Leino, 1998; Plant, Miller, Plant, & Nichol, 1994).

"Different drinking patterns give rise to very different health outcomes in different population groups. Both quantity and frequency are crucial variables in determining health risks" (WHO, 2003). For example, a person drinking 14 drinks a week at the rate of 2 each day with his supper at home is likely to experience a different set of outcomes than the person who also consumes 14 drinks, but confines them all to the weekend when he is celebrating with his friends and may need to drive. Understanding how individuals drink not only predicts what their risks might be, but also allows a more tightly targeted approach to managing these risks.

Taking its cue from the successful approaches implemented in the drug field, alcohol policy has been increasing its reliance on minimizing harm. The fundamental view inherent in this approach is that risks are intrinsic to all human activities. It is therefore necessary to recognize that although risks persist, they can be managed and reduced. In the case of alcohol consumption, the aim of such an approach is not to eliminate or even severely curtail drinking. Instead, it is to ensure that when people drink, they do so in as safe a manner as possible, and that their drinking environment is not conducive to harm.

Harm-reduction approaches allow interventions to be designed specifically for those particularly at risk without affecting the behaviors and choices of others whose drinking does not place them at risk for harm. A clear distinction exists between vulnerability and risk. "People are at risk if something negative might happen. People are vulnerable when, if something negative happens, it will damage them; vulnerability is defined by the damage, not the risk" (Spicker, 2001, p. 24). Vulnerability can be defined as the absence of protection and generally applies to those who are not within the mainstream of the general population for one reason or another, be it age, special health, or social conditions. Thus, it is necessary to design approaches that will provide protective measures for these populations above and beyond the measures that are crafted with the rest of the population in mind. Harm reduction offers the flexibility to do just that.

With regard to alcohol consumption, several potentially vulnerable populations have been identified and are the focus of specialized approaches. For example, pregnant women are considered vulnerable to certain drinking patterns, as are young people, the elderly, those with particular health problems that may be adversely affected by drinking, those with a particular genetic predisposition to alcohol dependence or the inability to metabolize alcohol, indigenous populations, and those who are otherwise excluded from the mainstream of society. It has also been suggested that those living in developing countries are particularly vulnerable because of changing drinking patterns and conditions within the alcohol market, although their vulnerability is attributable to a broad range of complex interactions.

The harm-reduction approach attempts to incorporate education and the provision of information in its overall strategy to equip individuals with the tools necessary to make informed decisions about drinking patterns and potential outcomes (Plant & Plant, 1997). Strategies for doing this were addressed in Chapter 4 on risk communication. Education about alcohol and drinking patterns can be found in a variety of forms, ranging from campaigns to educate the general public about alcohol content and drink sizes by labeling containers (Stockwell & Single, 1997) to measures specifically designed to educate consumers about drinking and driving. Specially tailored education or reminder measures have also been targeted at vulnerable populations and those particularly at risk. For example, pregnant women are the focus of health warning labels on containers of beverage alcohol in a number of countries (Greenfield, 1997; ICAP, 1997).

Official guidelines that are intended to provide information about alcohol consumption have been developed in a number of countries, based on the available scientific and medical evidence. Information included in these guidelines is aimed both at the general population and at groups that are particularly vulnerable. For, example, such guidelines address levels of drinking and limits associated with low risk (ICAP, 2003), providing separate information for men and women, as well as particular caveats. The need to address individual patterns is also increasingly addressed in the development of risk-reduction guidelines.

The current Australian Alcohol Guidelines offer information relevant to a range of individuals whose risks are likely to be different when it comes to alcohol consumption (Australian Government, 2002). Information is given separately for men and women, for the elderly and young people, and expressed in terms of daily and weekly consumption patterns. In addition, drinking patterns are related to the potential risk level associated with them, as listed in Table 6.1. *Low Risk* is defined as levels at which risk is minimal and benefits may exist for some individuals. *Risky* is characterized as the level at which risk for harm is significantly increased beyond any possible benefits. *High Risk* is defined as levels at which a substantial risk exists for serious harm and above which the risk increases rapidly.

An international survey of policymakers responsible for decisions about alcohol issues showed that among those who responded education about alcohol was considered the main priority in the development of alcohol policies (ICAP, 2003). Eighty-five percent of those surveyed cited this as a key goal. This issue headed the list for respondents from countries in both the developed and the developing world. Currently, alcohol education efforts through official

TABLE 6.1 Australian Alcohol Guidelines. Levels of
Short- and Long-Term Harm,
as Measured by Number of Standard Drinks[a]

For Risk of Acute Harm (in the short term)

MALES	Low Risk	Risky	High Risk
On any one day	Up to 6 on any one day	7 to 10 on any one day	11 or more on any one day
	No more than 3 days per week		

FEMALES	Low Risk	Risky	High Risk
On any one day	Up to 4 on any one day	5 to 6 on any one day	7 or more on any one day
	No more than 3 days per week		

For Risk of Chronic Harm (in the long term)

MALES	Low Risk	Risky	High Risk
On an average day	Up to 4 per day	5 to 6 per day	7 or more per day
Overall weekly level	Up to 28 per week	29 to 42 per week	43 or more per week

FEMALES	Low Risk	Risky	High Risk
Overall average day	Up to 2 per day	3 to 4 per day	5 or more per day
Overall weekly level	Up to 14 per week	15 to 28 per week	29 or more per week

[a]A standard drink in Australia is defined as the equivalent of 10 g of ethanol (National Alcohol Strategy, 2003).

governmental or quasi-governmental entities have been implemented in 25% of responding countries. Specialized education measures, such as those aimed exclusively at young people, are somewhat more widespread and have been implemented in 33% of the countries that responded to the survey.

A wide range of other harm-reduction measures exists, each with a different specific target audience. Designated driver programs, for example, have been used effectively to reduce the risk of drunk-driving accidents, particularly in relation to licensed premises where individuals may be offered incentives to refrain from drinking. This measure falls into the category of "responsible hospitality," as does training of servers in drinking establishments to recognize excessive and risky drinking behaviors among patrons, thus minimizing the potential for harm. Other similar measures in bars have been aimed at reducing the potential for violence through environmental modification (Graham & Homel, 1997). Poor ventilation, inadequate seating, loud noise, and the availability of glass that may be used as a weapon all create potential risks around certain drinking behaviors and can be modified for the purposes of harm reduction.

Cheaper than an ambulance, better than the morgue.

Wet shelters that have been set up in Canada as a measure to provide an alternative to heavy alcohol abuse by dependent individuals who are relying on non-potable forms of alcohol to satisfy their cravings and might easily end up dying on the street. The alcohol provided is cheap, paid for by the state, and provided in limited quantities—rationed, so those drinking it can be weaned. Without the shelters, they would be drinking mouthwash, rubbing alcohol, or vanilla, or they would be stoned on glue or aerosol.

The residents brew the alcohol themselves. They stay out of the emergency rooms. "Nearly 500 guys have been through the program since November 1996. Some have cleaned up completely. Some have moved on to nursing homes. Some have died; they'd have died anyway. Along the way, they've all had access to things they did not have on the street: doctors, nurses, cousellors" (Fiorito, 2002).

Alcohol poses a potential problem for particular groups of individuals. For various reasons, these individuals may either have an intrinsic biological vulnerability to alcohol (ICAP, 2001) or may be alcohol dependent. For them, the risks associated with alcohol consumption are higher than they are for the general population. The drinking patterns of these individuals merit particular attention and require approaches to risk management that may not be useful for the public.

Measures have been developed that allow the identification of those individuals for whom drinking is particularly problematic, as well as measures that seek to modify harmful drinking behaviors. Developed by WHO, the Alcohol Use Disorders Identification Test (AUDIT) has been used to identify problem drinkers (Saunders, Aasland, Amundsen, & Grant, 1993). When followed by brief intervention and counseling sessions, this approach is highly effective in changing problematic drinking patterns, as well as reducing health problems (Fleming et al., 2002). Programs aimed at identifying and modifying harmful drinking behaviors can be applied across cultures and settings and appear to be effective not only for adults, but also in changing the behaviors and potential risks for young people (Chung, Colby, Barnett, & Monti, 2002). Another harm-reduction approach that is aimed at the vulnerable group of alcohol-dependent individuals has been implemented in Australia. Commercially available flour used for baking and cooking is supplemented with the amino acid thiamine. Although the supplement has no effect on those who are not alcohol-dependent, it is effective in counteracting some of the symptoms of Wernicke–Korsakoff Syndrome in those who are (Ma & Truswell, 1995).

Alcohol Industry Efforts

A significant and expanding role exists for the private sector in the management of risk. Corporate social responsibility has led to various efforts to reduce risk in areas as diverse as supporting clean water initiatives, ensuring employee safety, and focusing on product integrity. Although the requirements of good corporate citizenship must be balanced against an industry's profit margin and demands of shareholders, the private sector recognizes that social responsibility is also good business practice.

Similar to other industries, producers of beverage alcohol have invested considerable resources into initiatives to reduce potential for risk to consumers through harm-reduction approaches. Consumer education is a high priority to raise awareness of positive and negative drinking patterns through campaigns and initiatives. Other initiatives include on-premise risk management through responsible service. Targeted interventions to reduce potential risk for harm are directed particularly at reducing drinking and driving and alcohol misuse by vulnerable groups, particularly young people. Although the producers of beverage alcohol or their associated organizations largely fund these initiatives, many are built on partnerships involving governments, communities, and civil society institutions, as well as joint ventures with partners from the private sector or research and educational institutions.

In order to facilitate and coordinate these activities, social aspects organizations (SAOs) have been established in a number of countries around the world. They exist primarily in countries in North America and Western Europe, but efforts are currently under way to set up additional SAOs in transitional economies and developing countries. SAOs focus primarily on drinking and driving and on educating young people about responsible drinking (Houghton, 1999). In addition to funding SAO activities, alcohol producers support similar initiatives through the direct involvement of their own companies and through trade associations in individual countries that represent the beer, wine, or distilled spirits sector.

Industry-sponsored interventions often rely on public campaigns and programs to deter drinking and driving. These include free taxi rides for bar and restaurant patrons whose ability to drive may be impaired, as well as designated-driver programs. The award-winning "I'll be Des" (Anti Drink–Drive DESignated Driver) Campaign, developed and implemented by The Portman Group, an SAO in the United Kingdom, is one such example. According to The Portman Group, "Des is aimed particularly at 18- to 40-year-old male drivers who constitute the group most at risk of being involved, injured, or killed in a drink–drive accident" (The Portman Group, 2003a). Similar campaigns have been integrated into social settings and entertainment venues for young people. The "Night-Rider" program, an effective initiative sponsored by the German brewers' association (Deutscher Brauer-Bund, 2003), is profiled in discos and other venues where there is likely to be a large target audience of young people and where drinking may also get out of hand.

Training programs aimed at those involved in the sale and serving of alcohol have been implemented effectively in several countries. These approaches are designed to educate staff at serving establishments to recognize intoxication among patrons and to manage risks associated with drinking by being vigilant of their patrons' consumption patterns and behaviors. These programs are generally carried out in partnership with retailers and licensed premises, as well as with community organizations and government. In some countries, these training programs are voluntary and may be implemented not only to reduce harm, but also potential legal liability. In others, these are mandatory and may be a condition for obtaining and retaining a server license.

Finally, many campaigns are designed to discourage drinking by those below the legal drinking age and to educate those above the limit about responsible practices. The Century Council, a U.S.-based SAO, has developed a number of approaches to both issues. Their "Cops in Shops" program, for example, is aimed at deterring the purchase of alcohol by individuals who are under the legal age, and it relies on the presence of undercover police officers and the participation of retailers. Materials have also been developed to assist parents in discussing drinking with their children, and training materials and curriculum guides crafted with the assistance of key educators are available to extend alcohol education into schools and onto university campuses (The Century Council, 2003). Similar industry-sponsored efforts are underway in other countries around the world, through SAOs, as well as through companies, their trade associations, and other entities.

An Integrative Approach to Alcohol Policy

The harm-reduction approach to risk management policy has two great strengths:

1. It is pragmatic, recognizing that risks are ubiquitous and inherent in virtually every behavior in which we engage. Furthermore, risky behavior is

not likely to be eliminated because, for many individuals, riskiness itself holds great appeal. Although we cannot do away with risks altogether, it is possible to manage them and to make many behaviors and situations considerably safer.
2. It is not proprietary in nature. In other words, no single entity or sector of society need be in total control of its implementation.

In fact, the harm-reduction approach has shown itself to be stronger and more effective when it involves multiple partners, all working toward a common goal. Unlike control measures, harm reduction is not restrictive; all those involved—government, the private sector, and the public itself—can assume ownership in its implementation.

Criteria for an integrative and comprehensive approach to alcohol policy based on harm reduction can be summarized as follows. These criteria call for the policy to be:

1. *Pragmatic:* based on facts rather than on beliefs
2. *Realistic:* recognizing that alcohol consumption is an integral part of many societies with both negative and positive effects
3. *Nonjudgmental:* realizing that those with alcohol-related problems or those who cause them should not be condemned
4. *Aimed at empowerment:* strengthening individual responsibility along with measures involving external controls
5. *Inclusive:* actively involving individuals and the community in policy development rather than having issues "addressed" only by those who hold positions of authority
6. *Synergystic:* stimulating cooperation and respect among all stakeholders and recognizing that differences are challenges, not obstacles (Buning, Gorgulho, Melcop, & O'Hare, 2003).

It is important to realize that a successful approach to alcohol policy and risk management relies on the integration of many elements and measures that have been discussed in this chapter. Government clearly plays an important role, and an appropriate degree of regulatory oversight and control are necessary to make the world a safer place. At the same time, a broader and more inclusive approach that extends beyond government alone (be it at the local, national, or global level) is likely to meet with greater success.

Public–Private Partnerships

Public–private partnerships are receiving increasing attention within the public health field. For example, when it comes to preventing disease, developing new drugs, or reducing the potential for harm associated with a range of products and behaviors, partnerships are becoming increasingly significant.

Nevertheless, considerable disagreement exists about the nature of public–private partnerships, the parameters that should define them, which entities may legitimately be included as partners, and whether partnerships are effective or desirable. The views on these complex issues fall into two basic camps. Certain individuals, in focusing on the "public–private" aspects of partnership, stress that the goals of the two sectors are inherently at odds and fundamentally incompatible with one another. Others focus on the notion of "partnership" itself, which "implies a commitment to a common goal through the joint provision of complementary resources and expertise, and the joint sharing of risks involved" (Ridley, 2001). Although negotiations and clear ground rules are necessary to ensure that partnerships actually work and to define the playing field and respective responsibilities, the concept of partnership implies that negotiations will tend in a positive instead of a negative direction.

Many public–private partnerships that exist involve commercial enterprise, the public sector, and civil society organizations. Within the health field, the objectives of such partnerships have been described by Widdus (2001), particularly with respect to efforts aimed at managing infectious diseases through the development of pharmaceuticals and vaccines. These objectives include developing and distributing products, strengthening health services, educating the public, improving product quality and regulation, and coordinating multifaceted efforts.

Many examples of successful partnership approaches to risk management in the health field are available. One such example is the Global Alliance for Vaccines and Immunization (GAVI). An international coalition, GAVI involves the active participation of intergovernmental organizations— WHO, the United Nations Children's Fund (UNICEF), the World Bank; national governments; philanthropic institutions; the public sector through the International Federation of Pharmaceutical Manufacturers Associations (IFPMA); research and public health institutions. The mission of the alliance is to garner resources for immunization and to channel these to developing countries. Within this partnership, each member has an equally important role to play.

It is important to recognize that the private and public sectors are motivated by different reasons and that these differences may be reflected in their involvement in partnerships. These motivations should be accepted for what they are: neither good nor bad, only different and inherent in the very nature of the two sectors. Thus, it is possible to focus on the end goal, which is the greater public good and benefits that the partnerships will bring. Perhaps it is less important *why* partnerships are created than the fact that they *are* created and *are* feasible and viable.

Public–private partnerships in the alcohol field, which share many of the objectives outlined in this section, are receiving greater attention. The alcohol industry, particularly producers, is playing a more prominent role in policy initiatives. Public education about the responsible use of beverage alcohol has been an important objective of these partnerships, supported by efforts to improve quality and self-regulation. The efforts of the beverage alcohol industry and its related organizations have been severely criticized by some in the public health field as disingenuous attempts to expand the alcohol market. To many of these critics, the alcohol industry, no matter what it does, will always remain a wolf in sheep's clothing, and its partnership efforts to manage risks will not be judged on their merits but discarded a priori as suspect and generally unacceptable (McCreanor, Casswell, & Hill, 2000). This position reflects an extreme point of view that is present in the public health field in general and is based less on fact than on ideology. Fortunately, there exists a broader and more open view that recognizes that the world is changing, that policies cannot remain entrenched in the status quo, and that when it comes to managing risks, partnerships between the private and public sectors are a useful tool and a sign of evolving approaches to policy. To obtain lasting and satisfactory results, it is far more practical to involve all relevant players than to exclude them.

Partnerships also carry caveats. Partnerships are not a panacea. Parallel but independent efforts by both the private and public sectors—as well as by the nongovernmental, educational, and health sectors—are also required and should be strengthened. Partnerships are most effective in situations where independent action has limited impact, where desired goals and terms of reference can be agreed by all parties, where expertise of each partner is complementary to the others, and where benefits to all those involved are clear and attainable. In addition, all those involved must contribute a reasonable balance of resources and expertise. Finally, partnerships must be carried out in the spirit of complete transparency if they are to succeed.

Effective partnerships exist around risk management and alcohol. Many of the efforts initiated by SAOs, for example, rely on partnerships with the community and institutions to be effective. Often, government is involved. In Southern Africa, for example, an industry–government partnership was responsible for the development of an integrative and effective approach to alcohol education in the face of considerable odds. Where the attrition rate at elementary schools is higher than 50% and a large proportion of children grow up without parents or an intact family structure, students need to be equipped with skills that will allow them to make responsible choices in life. These decisions cover many aspects of social conduct, including drinking.

In a joint effort involving national and regional governments, the education sector and nongovernmental organizations, the beverage alcohol industry has for several years sponsored an ongoing program called "Growing Up" to teach life skills to schoolchildren in South Africa and Botswana (ICAP, 2000a). According to an evaluation of the program, it has achieved considerable success in changing behavior. The beverage alcohol industry within the region was actively involved in the design, implementation, and funding of this project and the production of materials to support it. Growing Up is now an integral part of the curriculum in a number of government regional schools.

Partnerships mean that multiple sectors can be involved in addressing specific issues within a broad context and alongside other related issues. A notable example is that the alcohol industry is one of many partners in the Global Road Safety Partnership (GRSP). This initiative, involving the International Federation of Red Cross and Red Crescent Societies (IFRC), the World Bank, governmental and civic organizations, nongovernmental organizations, and a wide range of private sector institutions, is aimed at increasing road safety and reducing the risk of traffic crashes and deaths, particularly in developing countries and transition economies. Although alcohol is a focus, it is addressed within the context of many issues to create a comprehensive and integrated approach to minimizing road hazards. As a result, whereas the beverage alcohol industry is an actively engaged partner, so are the automotive and petrochemical industries, the insurance industry, and others with a stake in road safety, each contributing its own part in order to present a combined strategy.

These examples of public–private partnerships describe how risk management endeavors can be effectively implemented in a range of contexts. Whether the approach is broad, with alcohol playing only a small part within a larger context, or whether the focus is centered on alcohol-related risks, public–private partnerships hold significant promise for the future and bring together resources and experience that otherwise might not be available.

Alcohol Policy Responses and Developing Countries

Much of the preceding discussion of policy development is perhaps most relevant to developed countries in which government and civil society institutions are well established and where resources are plentiful. The majority of the world's population, however, lives in countries that are undergoing or have recently undergone social, political, and economic changes. In these countries, institutions and a framework within which to effectively address alcohol issues are often lacking. Whereas alcohol problems may be a significant public health concern in many developing countries, they may not be a high priority on the national health agenda. Alcohol policies, where they explicitly exist, may be subsumed under general health programs and take second place to communicable diseases, nutrition issues, the aftermath of natural disasters, and other concerns.

The results of a 2002 survey of key policy makers in the alcohol field were analyzed to determine differences between mature and emerging markets with regard to alcohol policies currently in existence (ICAP, 2002). The analysis shows that among the emerging market countries that responded to the survey, the most common policy measures had to do with licensing, but that other measures geared at education and various harm-reduction approaches were not widely implemented. The survey also suggested, however, that policy measures that addressed education of consumers and of high-risk groups, such as young people, were among the top priorities for future policy development both in mature and emerging markets. (see Table 6.2).

Although the potential risks surrounding alcohol consumption and the resulting problems may be well known in developing countries, there often exists a dearth of systematic information about prevailing drinking patterns (Grant, Houghton, & Kast, 1998; Haworth & Simpson, 2004; Riley & Marshall, 1999; Room et al., 2002) as well as the extent to which different outcomes can be found within the population. Because drinking patterns are considered as intrinsically linked to social variables (Rehm et al., 1996), a thorough understanding of drinking patterns offers insight into how alcohol is consumed, its meaning within a particular cultural and social context, the risks and benefits associated with its consumption, and the policies needed to minimize risk and ensure the well-being of the community as well as individuals.

A wide diversity exists in the attitudes that prevail in developing countries with regard to the place of alcohol in society. Traditional views on alcohol consumption, along with traditional beverages are being displaced in some areas by a "Western" style of drinking and the consumption of commercial alcohol. These are often manifestations of broader changes

TABLE 6.2 Existing Alcohol Policies in Mature and Emerging Markets

Policy	Mature Markets (% of responses)	Emerging Markets (% of responses)
Drunk driving	100	69
Minimum legal drinking age	81	53
Licensing	81	72
Advertising and promotion	56	41
Guidelines	44	22
Alcohol education (youth)	38	31
Server training	38	0
Alcohol education (general)	25	22
Health warning labels	13	28

Source: From ICAP, 2002. *Industry views on beverage alcohol advertising and marketing, with special reference to young people.* Retrieved from http://www.icap.org. With permission.

occurring in many societies. Occurring mostly in urban areas, these new drinking patterns offer a contrast between the ritual and often-therapeutic function of traditional beverages and imported beverages as a status symbol and expression of social and economic success (Heath, 1998). Rural drinking patterns, on the other hand, are still largely characterized by the consumption of noncommercial and locally produced alcohol and traditional beverages (Grant, 1998; Haworth & Simpson, 2004; Heath, 2000 Room et al., 2002).

Social norms and structures occupy an especially prominent place when it comes to alcohol in developing countries. Alcohol plays a central and varied role in traditional social interaction, and its production is frequently integrated into everyday life. In developing countries, a large proportion of beverage alcohol is still made in traditional ways. Home brew is accountable for an estimated 30% of consumption in Sri Lanka, 80% in Tanzania, and 50% in India (Heath, 1998). In addition, in many developing countries, abstention rates are high, especially among women, and alcohol consumption may be confined to rituals and special occasions (ICAP, 2000b). In Jamaica, for example, the abstention rate is 68% of the total population, and 80% of Jamaican women are reported as abstaining from alcohol. In Guatemala, 52% of people are abstainers, while in Sri Lanka this figure is 70%.

Thus, the question of how to address alcohol policies in developing countries and emerging markets is a complex one, especially when it comes to risk. Blanket approaches used elsewhere, for example in Scandinavian countries or within North America, may not be appropriate within the context of developing countries. Novel approaches are called for, approaches based on an understanding of the role of alcohol within a particular society, including its symbolism and cultural meaning. The nature of the risks that are related to alcohol in developing areas of the world is also different from the risks that may be present in mature economies. For example, the risk of workplace consequences may not be as high in developing countries; however, the risk for familial problems and the effects of drained family resources are extremely high. As discussed in Chapter 2, the basic perception of risk may also be culture-specific, requiring it to be addressed in a culture-specific way.

As Heath (1998) points out,

- Without a good understanding of the norms of a population, it is difficult to make early identification of individuals who are at high risk for many kinds of alcohol-related problems or who are showing early signs that such problems may develop.
- Similarly, a great many drinking problems in any population defy diagnosis unless one is familiar with cultural norms and expectations.
- Among the several approaches to treatment that are available, some are appropriate to members of one culture but not another.

The same holds true of broader alcohol policy measures aimed at reducing risk.

In light of the relatively low priority given to alcohol issues by governments of many developing countries where concerns and resources are directed elsewhere, policy approaches must often rely more heavily on other players in the alcohol arena to minimize potential risk for harm. Here, civil society organizations can play a crucial role. For example, in several Central and Eastern European countries and former Soviet states, the Soros Foundation and Open Society Institute are actively engaged in developing approaches for harm reduction in the alcohol field (Stefan Batory Foundation, 2003). Many of these ventures are carried out in partnership with other entities and are grounded in a pragmatic approach to harm reduction within a particular cultural setting.

The beverage alcohol industry also has a continuing role in helping to manage risks involving alcohol in developing countries. For example, partnerships have been created with police forces in a number of countries to monitor the trade in illicit and counterfeit alcohol. Testing kits have been developed that can help ensure that products are not contaminated and do not contain potentially harmful impurities. Another approach is the upholding of ethical standards with regard to sales and promotion of alcohol. These standards should be at least as high as they are in developed countries, and often higher, especially in the absence of government measures to ensure that self-regulatory codes are implemented and adhered to. Despite the existence of these examples, however, few efforts to promote responsible drinking practices and prevent alcohol misuse exist outside the developed world (Pedlow, 1998).

Efforts have been made to develop a framework within which the beverage alcohol industry can continue to contribute to responsible practices in developing countries. A *Suggested Framework for Responsibility* (Pedlow, 1998) offers a number of areas in which the beverage alcohol industry can be actively involved in risk management of its products in the developing world. Specific examples of such efforts include systematic efforts to obtain information about drinking patterns, alcohol education to promote responsible drinking, and promotional and marketing practices aimed at reducing risk.

SUMMARY

The success of promising efforts to develop future comprehensive policies aimed at managing risks associated with drinking is predicated upon a number of elements. They are inclusive, involving the public, private, and nongovernmental sectors, all of which have a legitimate stake and need to function as equal partners in formulating policy. The integrative approach to policy development extends beyond simply including diverse partners. It also entails adapting competing, and at times seemingly incompatible, policy elements—drawing from them valuable lessons and integrating them into an approach that is pragmatic and fair.

In practice, a comprehensive approach to managing risks involving alcohol, or any other issue, should be founded on solid science to assess the true nature of the risks involved and the options that are presented. This assessment should include a realistic picture of costs and benefits, reflecting the economic feasibility of various risk management alternatives. Risk management policy should also be well grounded in the legal system, taking into account legislation and reasonable regulatory options.

Integrative policy approaches cannot overstress the role of the public—the individuals who will ultimately be affected by whatever decisions are made and policies implemented. This includes weighing the public's sensitivity to risk and the degree to which it believes in the credibility of risk management options. As previous chapters have discussed, not all sources of information about risk are equally credible. In addition, the public needs to be involved in decisions and should have access to full and accurate information, especially about the extent of the risks and the options for their management. Finally, the political importance of risk and the acceptability of options must also be weighed within the context of culture, values, and perceptions.

Policy approaches to minimizing the risks related to alcohol require the application of a range of strategies, executed through an inclusive and integrated approach. Among the essential elements of an effective public policy are an appropriate degree of control over access to alcohol, communication of the best available information to consumers and health professionals about potential harms and risks associated with inappropriate drinking patterns, recognition of the importance of minimizing the risks associated with a variety of drinking patterns, occasions, and other special circumstances.

REFERENCES

Aichmayer, S., & Schindler, I. (2002, May 15). *The precautionary principle—A necessary complement to impact based approaches.* Presentation at the SETAC Conference, Challenges in Environmental Risk Assessment and Modelling: Linking Basic and Applied Research, Vienna, Austria.

Annan, K. (1998). Address to World Economic Forum [Speech]. Retrieved August, 21 2002 from http://www.un.org/partners/business/davos.htm.

Australian Broadcasting Corporation: News Online. (2003, November 11). *Duty-free craze spreads across Finland, Sweden.* Retrieved November 18 2003, from http://www.abc.net.au/ news/indepth/featureitems/s986833.htm.

Australian Government. (2002). *Australian Alcohol Guidelines.* Canberra: Department of Health and Ageing, Population Health Division.

Baker, T. K., Johnson, M. B., Voas, R. B., & Lange, J. E. (2000). Reduce youthful binge drinking: Call an election in Mexico. *Journal of Safety Research, 31,* 61–69.

Beane, E. A., & Beck, J. C. (1991). Court based civil commitment of alcoholics and substance abusers. *Bulletin of the American Academy of Psychiatry and the Law,* 359–366.

Buning, E., Gorgulho, M., Melcop, A. G., & O'Hare, P. (Eds.). (2003). *Alcohol and harm reduction: An innovative approach for communities in transition.* Amsterdam: International Coalition on Alcohol and Harm Reduction.

Byrne, J. (2002). *Alcohol retail monopolies.* Retrieved from http://www.icap.org/invited/opinion_byrne.html.

Center for Substance Abuse Prevention/International Center for Alcohol Policies. (1998). *What do others hear when we speak about alcohol?* Working Papers. Washington, DC: Author.

The Century Council. (2003). Retrieved from http://www.centurycouncil.org.

Chung, T., Colby, S. M., Barnett, N. P., & Monti, P. M. (2002). Alcohol Use Disorders Identification Test: Factor structure in an adolescent emergency department sample. *Alcoholism: Clinical and Experimental Research, 26,* 223–231.

De Sadeleer, N. (2002). *Environmental principles: From political slogans to legal rules.* Oxford, UK: Oxford University Press.

Deutscher Brauer-Bund. (2003). *Night-Rider.* Retrieved August 21, 2003, from http://www.night-rider.org/nightrider.html.

Duffy, M. (1991). Advertising and the consumption of tobacco and alcoholic drink: A system-wide analysis. *Scottish Journal of Political Economy, 38,* 369–385.

Duffy, M. (1995). Advertising in demand systems for alcoholic drinks and tobacco: A comparative study. *Journal of Policy Modeling, 17,* 557–577.

Edwards, G., Anderson, P., Babor, T. F., Casswell, S., Ferrence, R., Giesbrecht, N., et al. (1994). *Alcohol policy and the public good.* New York: Oxford University Press.

Edwards, R., & Glover, J. (2001). Risk, citizenship and welfare: Introduction. In R. Edwards & J. Glover (Eds.), *Risk and citizenship: Key issues in welfare* (pp. 1–18). London: Routledge.

European Commission. (1999. February 17). *Communication from the Commission to the Council concerning the employment aspects of the decision to abolish tax- and duty-free sales for intra-community travellers.* Brussels: Author.

European Policy Center. (1999) *The politicisation of science and the precautionary principle.* Brussels: Author.

Fiorito, J. (2002, July 2). *Cheaper than an ambulance, better than the morgue.* Retreived from http://www.globeandmail.com (Globe and Mail).

Fisher, J. C. (1993). *Advertising, alcohol consumption, and abuse: A worldwide survey.* Westport, CT: Greenwood Press.

Fisher, J. C., & Cook, P. A. (1995). *Advertising, alcohol consumption, and mortality: An empirical investigation.* Westport, CT: Greenwood Press.

Fleming, C. M., & Manson, S. M. (1990). Native American women. In R. C. Engs (Ed.), *Women: Alcohol and other drugs* (pp. 143–148). Dubuque: Kendall/Hunt Publishing Company.

Fleming, M. F., Mundt, M. P., French, M. T., Manwell, L. B., Stauffacher, E. A., & Barry, K. L. (2002). Brief physician advice for problem drinkers: Long-term efficacy and benefit-cost analysis. *Alcoholism: Clinical and Experimental Research, 26,* 36–43.

Franklin, J. (Ed.). (1998). *The politics of risk society.* Cambridge, UK: Polity Press.

Goel, R. K., & Morey, M. J. (1995) The interdependence of cigarette and liquor demand. *Southern Economic Journal, 62,* 451–459.

Gordon, A. J., Wentz, C. M., Gibbon, J. L., Mason, A. D., Freyder, P. J., & O'Toole, T. P. (2001). Relationships between patient characteristics and unsuccessful substance abuse detoxification. *Journal of Addictive Diseases, 20,* 41–53.

Gorman, D. M., Speer, P. W., Gruenewald, P. J., & Labouvie, E. W. (2001). Spatial dynamics of alcohol availability, neighborhood structure and violent crime. *Journal of Studies on Alcohol, 62,* 628–636.

Graham, K., & Homel, R. (1997). Creating safer bars. In M. Plant, E. Single, & T. Stockwell (Eds.), *Alcohol: Minimising the harm. What works?* (pp. 171–192). London: Free Association Books.

Grant, M. (Ed.). (1998). *Alcohol and emerging markets: Patterns, problems and responses.* Philadelphia, PA: Brunner/Mazel.

Grant, M., Houghton, E., & Kast, J. (1998). Drinking patterns and policy development. In M. Grant (Ed.), *Alcohol and emerging markets: Patterns, problems and responses* (pp. 1–17). Philadelphia, PA: Brunner/Mazel.

Grant, M., & Litvak, J. (Eds). (1998). *Drinking patterns and their consequences.* Washington, DC: Taylor & Francis.

Greenfield, T. K. (1997). Warning labels: Evidence on harm reduction from long-term American surveys. In M. Plant, E. Single, & T. Stockwell (Eds.), *Alcohol: Minimising the harm. What works?* (pp. 105–125). London: Free Association Books.

Gruenewald, P. J., Johnson, F. W., & Treno, A. J. (2002). Outlets, drinking and driving: A multilevel analysis of availability. *Journal of Studies on Alcohol, 63,* 460–468.

Gruenewald, P. J., Russell, M., Light, J., Lipton, R., Searles, J., Johnson, F., et al. (2002). One drink to a lifetime of drinking: Temporal structures of drinking patterns. *Alcoholism: Clinical and Experimental Research, 26,* 916–925.

Haworth, A., & Simpson, R. (2004). *Moonshine markets: Issues in unrecorded beverage alcohol production and consumption.* New York: Brunner-Routledge.

Heath, D. B. (1998). Beverage alcohol in developing regions: An anthropological and epidemiological perspective on public health issues. In M. Grant (Ed.), *Alcohol and emerging markets: Patterns, problems and responses* (pp. 287–309). Philadelphia, PA: Brunner/Mazel.

Heath, D. B. (2000). *Drinking occasions: Comparative perspectives on alcohol and culture.* Philadelphia, PA: Brunner/Mazel.

Houghton, E. (1999). Comparative analysis of alcohol education programs sponsored by the beverage alcohol industry. *Journal of Alcohol and Drug Education, 43,* 15–33.

International Center for Alcohol Policies (ICAP). (1997). *Health warning labels* (Report No. 3). Washington, DC: Author.

ICAP. (1998). *Drinking Age Limits* (Report No. 4, revised 2002). Washington, DC: Author.

ICAP. (2000a). *Life skills education in South Africa and Botswana.* Washington, DC: Author.

ICAP. (2000b). *Who are the abstainers?* (Report No. 8). Washington, DC: Author.

ICAP. (2001). *Self-regulation of beverage alcohol advertising* (Report No. 9). Washington, DC: Author.

ICAP. (2002). *Industry views on beverage alcohol advertising and marketing, with special reference to young people.* Retrieved from http://www.icap.org.

ICAP. (2003). *Alcohol policy through partnership: Is the glass half-empty or half-full? An international survey of policy makers.* Washington, DC: Author.

Joensen, D. (2002). *Alcohol retail monopolies.* Retrieved from http://www.icap.org/invited/opinion_joensen.html.

Kingsley, W. L. (1871, April). The blue laws. *The New Englander and Yale Review, 243–304.*

Ledermann, S. (1952). Une mortalité d'origine économique en France: La mortalité d'origine ou d'appoint. *Semaine Medicale, 28,* 418–421.

Ledermann, S., & Tabah, F. (1951). Nouvelles donnees sur la mortalité d'origine alcoolique. *Population, G,* 41–56.

Lyall, S. (2003, October 13). *Something cheap in the state of Denmark: Liquor.* Retrieved from http://www.newyorktimes.com.

Ma, J. J., & Truswell, A. S. (1995). Wernicke–Korsakoff Syndrome in Sydney hospitals: Before and after thiamine enrichment of flour. *Medical Journal of Australia, 163,* 531–534.

Manning, W. G., Blumberg, L., & Moulton, L. H. (1995). The demand for alcohol: The differential response to price. *Journal of Health Economics, 14,* 123–148.

McCreanor, T., Casswell, S., & Hill, L. (2000). ICAP and the perils of partnership. *Addiction, 95,* 185.

Miller, J. D. (1987). Scientific literacy in the United States. In D. Evered & M. O'Connor (Eds.), *Communicating science to the public* (pp. 19–40). Chichester, UK: John Wiley & Sons.

Morris, J. (2000). Defining the precautionary principle. In Morris, J. (Ed.), *Rethinking risk and the precautionary principle* (pp. 1–21). Oxford, UK: Butterworth-Heinemann.

Moss, D. A. (2002). *When all else fails: Government as the ultimate risk manager.* Cambridge, MA: Harvard University Press.

National Alcohol Strategy. (2003). *Drinking patterns and levels of risk,* Fact Sheet 18. Canberra, Australia: Department of Health and Ageing, Population Health Division.

Nelson, J. P. (1997). *Broadcast advertising and U.S./demand for alcoholic beverages: System-wide estimates with quarterly data.* Washington, DC: Federal Trade Commission.

Nelson, J. P., & Moran, J. R. (1995). Advertising and U.S. alcoholic beverage demand: System-wide estimates. *Applied Economics, 27,* 1225–1236.

Norström, T., & Skog, O. J. (2003). Saturday opening of alcohol retail shops in Sweden: An impact analysis. *Journal of Studies on Alcohol, 64,* 393–401.

Österberg, E., & Karlsson, T. (2002). Alcohol policies in EU member states. *The Globe, 1,* 12–13.

Pedlow G. (1998). *A suggested framework for responsibility.* Washington, DC: International Center for Alcohol Policies.

Perkins, H. W., & Craig, D. W. (2002). *A multifaceted social norms approach to high-risk drinking: Lessons from Hobart and William Smith Colleges.* Newton, MA: The Higher Education Center for Alcohol and Other Drug Prevention.

Plant, M. (2001). Learning by experiment. In E. Houghton & A.M. Roche (Eds.), *Learning about drinking* (pp. 129–146). Philadelphia: Brunner-Routledge.

Plant, M., Single, E., & Stockwell, T. (Eds.). (1997*). Alcohol: Minimising the harm. What works?* London: Free Association Books.

Plant, M. A., Miller, P., Plant, M. L., & Nichol, P. (1994). No such thing as a safe glass. *British Medical Journal, 308,* 6–7.

Plant, M. A., & Plant, M. L. (1997). Alcohol education and harm minimisation. In M. Plant, E. Single, & T. Stockwell (Eds.), *Alcohol: Minimising the harm. What works?* (pp. 193–210). London: Free Association Books.

The Portman Group. (2003a). *I'll be des.* Retrieved August 21, 2003, from http://www.portmangroup.org.uk/initiatives/drive.asp.

The Portman Group. (2003b). *Code of practice on the naming, packaging and promotion of alcoholic drinks* (3rd ed.). London: The Portman Group.

Rabinowitz, J., & Marjefsky, S. (1998). Alcohol and drug abuse: Predictors of being expelled from and dropping out of alcohol treatment. *Psychiatric Services, 49,* 187–189.

Rehm, J., Ashley, M. J., Room, R., Single, E., Bondy, S., Ferrence, R., et al. (1996). On the emerging paradigm of drinking patterns and their social and health consequences. *Addiction, 91,* 1615–1621.

Ridley, R. G. (2001). Putting the partnership into public–private partnership. *Bulletin of the World Health Organization, 79,* 694.

Riley, L., & Marshall, M. (1999). *Alcohol and public health in 8 developing countries* (Document No.: WHO/HSC/SAB/99.9). Geneva: World Health Organization.

Romanus, G. (2002). *Alcohol retail monopolies.* Retrieved from http://www.icap.org/invited/opinion_romanus.html.

Room, R. (2001, August 19–21). *Why have a retail alcohol monopoly?* Paper presented at an International Seminar on Alcohol Retail Monopolies, Harrisburg, PA.

Room, R., Jernigan, D., Carlini-Marlatt, B., Gureje, O., Mäkelä, K., Marshall, M., et al. (2002). *Alcohol in developing societies: A public health approach.* Helsinki: Finnish Foundation for Alcohol Studies in collaboration with the World Health Organization.

Saunders, J. B., Aasland, O. G., Amundsen, A., & Grant, M. (1993). Alcohol consumption and related problems among primary health care patients. WHO collaborative project on early detection of persons with harmful alcohol consumption—I. *Addiction, 88*(3), 349–362.

Saunders, J. B. & de Burgh, S. (1998). The distribution of alcohol consumption. In M. Grant & J. Litvak (Eds.), *Drinking patterns and their consequences* (pp. 129–152). Washington, DC: Taylor & Francis.

Sines, N. J., & Ekman, J. (1996). *The minimum drinking age and alcohol policy: An historical overview and response to the renewed debate in Wisconsin.* Resource Center Report, 96-1. Retrieved from http://www.law.wisc.edu/rcid/resourcecenter/ResourceReports/report0496.htm.

Single, E., & Leino, V. E. (1998). The levels, patterns, and consequences of drinking. In M. Grant & J. Litvak (Eds.), Drinking patterns and their consequences (pp. 7–24). Washington, DC: Taylor & Francis.

Sjöberg, L. (1998). World views, political attitudes and risk perception. *Risk: Health, Safety and Environment, 9,* 137–152.

Skog, O.-J. (2000). An experimental study of a change from over-the-counter to self-service sales of alcoholic beverages in monopoly outlets. *Journal of Studies on Alcohol, 61,* 95–100.

Slovic, P. (1990). Choice. In D. Osherson & E. Smith (Eds), *Thinking: An invitation to cognitive science,* Vol. 3. (pp. 89–116). Cambridge, MA: The MIT Press.

Smith, D. I. (1990). Consumption and advertising of alcoholic beverages in Australia, 1969–86. *Drug and Alcohol Review, 9,* 33–41.

Spicker, P. (2001). Social insecurity and social protection. In R. Edwards & J. Glover (Eds.), *Risk and citizenship: Key issues in welfare.* London: Routledge.

Stefan Batory Foundation. (2003). Retrieved August 20, 2003, from http://www.batory.org.pl/english/com/index.htm.

Stockwell, T., & Gruenewald, P. (2001). Controls on the physical availability of alcohol. In N. Heather, T. J. Peters, & T. Stockwell (Eds.), *International handbook of alcohol dependence and problems* (pp. 699–719). Chichester, UK: John Wiley & Sons Ltd.

Stockwell, T., & Single, E. (1997). Standard unit labelling of alcohol containers. In M. Plant, E. Single, & T. Stockwell (Eds.), *Alcohol: Minimising the harm. What works?* (pp. 85–104). London: Free Association Books.

Sweden v. European Commission. (2000). *Globe: International Alcohol and Drug Problems, 1,* 16–17.

Voas, R. B., Lange, J. E., & Johnson, M. B. (2002). Reducing high-risk drinking by young Americans south of the border: The impact of a partial ban on sales of alcohol. *Journal of Studies on Alcohol, 63,* 286–292.

The Warsaw Voice. (2002, March 31, No. 13). *Hangover for Newsweek.* Retrieved from http://www.warsawvoice.pl/v701/News06.html.

Wells, S., & Graham, K. (2003). Aggression involving alcohol: Relationship to drinking patterns and social context. *Addiction, 98,* 33–42.

Widdus, R. (2001). Public–private partnerships for health: Their main targets, their diversity, and their future directions. *Bulletin of the World Health Organization, 79,* 713–720.

World Health Organization. (WHO) (1993). *European alcohol action plan.* (Document No.: EUR/ICAP/ADA 035). Copenhagen: Author.

WHO. (1995). *European charter on alcohol.* Copenhagen: Author.

WHO. (2003). *Global alcohol database: Country data on alcohol.* Retrieved August 20, 2003, from http://www3.who.int/whosis/alcohol/alcohol_patterns_general.cfm?path=whosis,alcohol,alcoholpatterns,alcohol_patterns_general&language=english.

Index

Date Due

BRODART, CO.   Cat. No. 23-233-003   Printed in U.S.A.

REASONABLE RISK

International Center for Alcohol Policies
Series on Alcohol in Society